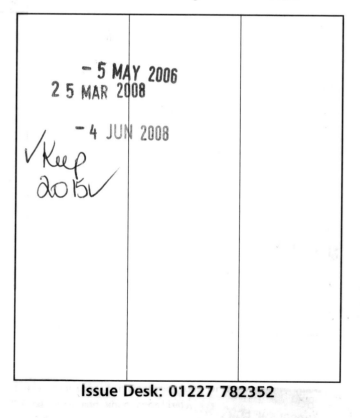

The reform of child care law

The Children Act 1989 introduces the most radical changes in child care law for a generation and will have significant effects on all professionals practising in this area.

Concentrating on fieldwork aspects of the new law – the definition of parental responsibilities, emergency powers, care and supervision orders, and court proceedings – *The Reform of Child Care Law* places the new act in its historical and political context and forms a concise, practical guide to the legislation. It will be invaluable, both for training and everyday reference, to social workers, health visitors, and to fieldworkers in community medicine, education, and other services with responsibilities for children.

The authors: John Eekelaar is a Fellow in Law at Pembroke College, Oxford and Robert Dingwall is a Research Fellow at Wolfson College and Centre for Socio-Legal Studies, University of Oxford. Together they have written and researched extensively about the workings of family and child care law. They were also involved in many of the informal discussions which led up to the drafting of the Children Act 1989.

The reform of child care law
A practical guide to the
Children Act 1989

John Eekelaar

and

Robert Dingwall

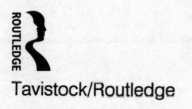

Tavistock/Routledge

First published 1990
by Routledge
11 New Fetter Lane, London EC4P 4EE

© 1990 John Eekelaar and Robert Dingwall

Typeset by NWL Editorial Services
Langport, Somerset TA10 9DG

Printed and bound in Great Britain by
Biddles Ltd, Guildford and King's Lynn

British Library Cataloguing in Publication Data

Eekelaar, John
The reform of child care law: a practical guide to the Children
Act 1989
1. Great Britain. Children. Care. Law
I. Title II. Dingwall, Robert
344.104'327

ISBN 0-415-01736-X

Contents

List of statutes

List of cases

Preface

The Children Act 1989 is the most comprehensive enactment on children in our legislative history. Some of the reforms which it introduces rewrite the very language used by generations of lawyers and child care professionals. Other changes are more subtle but will still have a significant impact on practice. No administrator, fieldworker or student of child care and child protection law and practice can avoid a fundamental reappraisal of existing habits and methods of working in the light of this new legislation.

The Act completed its passage through Parliament in 1989. However, many details, some significant, still have to be settled by rules and regulations made by ministers using powers conferred on them by the Act. It is likely to take at least a year before this process is complete and the Act is not expected to be implemented until autumn 1991. Until then, the "old" law will continue to apply. But, for ease of comprehension, we have written our text on the assumption that the Act has been brought fully into effect. When the Act is brought into operation, there will be special transitional arrangements to cover its effect on powers acquired previously. We have referred to these only in outline and would recommend fieldworkers to seek specialist guidance from the appropriate local authority department.

This book is primarily intended as a practical guide to child welfare and child protection law. For this reason we have dealt only very cursorily with those aspects of the Act whose effect is mainly administrative, like the changes in the registration and regulation of various facilities provided for children.

Throughout the book, the expression "the 1989 Act" refers to the Children Act 1989, and references to section numbers refer to sections of that Act unless stated to the contrary.

John Eekelaar
Robert Dingwall
November 1989

Chapter one

The historical background

The Children Act 1989 tries to create a uniform and coherent framework for strands in child welfare law which have developed largely independently of each other over some hundreds of years. In the short term, it was precipitated by the report of the Social Services Select Committee of the House of Commons in 1984, which we shall refer to as the *Select Committee Report*. Having conducted a series of hearings into the working of the law in disputes between public authorities and parents about the care or custody of children, the Committee concluded that the Government should undertake a thorough review of legislation and practice in this area.[1] The review was carried out by an interdepartmental working party of civil servants in co-operation with the Law Commission, an independent, though publicly funded, body responsible for monitoring the general development of the law. In October 1985 the working party issued a Consultative Document, *Review of Child Care Law* (referred to here as the *Review Report*) and in January 1987 the Government presented its response in a White Paper, *The Law on Child Care and Family Services* (here, the *White Paper*).[2]

Quite independently of the initiative of the Social Services Committee, the Law Commission had also announced in 1984 that, because of the confused legal position of children in private disputes about their care or custody, it would review this area of law.[3] Although the *Review Report* and the *White Paper* form the basis of most of the reforms described in this book, some of them result from the extensive work by the Law Commission since 1984.[4]

Public opinion, and some of the details of the legislation, may also have been influenced by the reports from various inquiries into supposed failures of the child protection system. The most important were the reports into the death of Jasmine Beckford (*A Child in Trust*) in 1985 (here, the *Jasmine Beckford Report*) and into the handling of alleged child sexual abuse in Cleveland in 1988 (here, the *Cleveland Report*). Other reports which achieved some prominence during this period included those into the deaths of Heidi Koseda (1985), Tyra Henry (1985) and Kimberley Carlile (1985).[5]

In order to understand the new legislation fully, however, it is necessary to sketch the historical processes which shaped the previous law and which brought about the demands for change. The old law, as we have said, was not uniform. Separate statutory provisions and systems of administration and adjudication had grown up in response to the different contexts in which children posed problems for the adult world. For the sake of convenience, we will organize these into four categories which we will call *child care law*, *child protection law*, the *wardship jurisdiction* and the *divorce jurisdiction*.

Child care law

Modern child care law is the successor of the Poor Law. The economic conditions of the sixteenth century created widespread unemployment and a population drifting in search of work. This put severe strain on the economic self-sufficiency of the rural family and on the ability of many adults to provide for the needs of their children. The Reformation had undermined the capacity of the Church to organize relief and the Poor Law developed as a secular substitute. Among other provisions, it led to the introduction of enforceable legal duties upon parents to provide for children who would otherwise be left destitute. It also empowered civil parish authorities to set to work or compulsorily apprentice those children whose parents could not help them. But, although many children presumably benefited from such policies, it does not seem that their own interests were primary concerns. The legal commentator Blackstone observed in 1765 that the purpose was that they might "render their abilities in their several stations of the greatest advantage to the commonwealth".[6]

This general approach to the problem of poor children changed little until the early nineteenth century. Much depended upon the individual decisions of each parish in response to particular cases. There was, however, growing criticism of other aspects of the Poor Law, which were felt to be an insufficient deterrent to idleness and indiscipline. In 1834 the system was reformed. The poor would receive assistance only if they entered a workhouse, where conditions would be harder than those experienced by the poorest wage earners. (This was known as the principle of "less eligibility".) In practice, there were never enough workhouse places in most areas and they tended to fill up with those whose poverty resulted from age, sickness, disability or mental incapacity. Although the drafters of the 1834 legislation had not intended that such people should be subjected to a punitive regime, the system remained until the twentieth century officially focused on deterring the able-bodied from falling into unemployment.

Inevitably, thousands of children, orphaned, deserted or simply members of the poorest families, found their way into the workhouses. By 1840 there were estimated to be over 64,000 of them. The general duties of the Poor Law authorities to secure their employment or apprenticeship remained essentially unchanged until 1948 and continued to influence legislation until the 1989 Act. Within this framework, though, there emerged a range of provisions which reflected changing perceptions of the rights of individuals, the role of families and the responsibilities of society.

These changes were first evident in the shift from using pauper children as a source of cheap labour to providing for their education and industrial training separately, if possible, from the workhouse. Although the principle of less eligibility was grounded in a severe view of human nature, viewing poverty as the result of individual moral weakness (although potentially correctable by a deterrent regime), contemporary philanthropists came to see destitution and its associate, delinquency, as socially caused. Their preferred solution lay in removing poor children from the corrupting influences around them and providing a morally wholesome environment. A number of philanthropic societies developed schemes for the "rescue" of poor children, although the Poor Law itself remained a battleground between their views and those of the advocates of less eligibility.

A critical constraint on improving conditions for workhouse children was the reluctance to give them any advantage over the children of the employed poor, by, for example, more generous educational opportunities. Once the Education Act 1870 created local education authorities with the major responsibility for schooling *all* the nation's children, the main function of the Poor Law shifted to

3

the provision of a home environment for those children in its care.

> [The Poor Law authorities] saw that variety was needed in the
> treatment of children, some responding to boarding-out, care in
> a scattered home or voluntary home, or finding their best hope
> of success in emigration. Much headway was made, and by the
> beginning of the twentieth century the new methods of care
> were being widely used. Of 69,030 in poor law care in 1908 less
> than a third were in workhouses or infirmaries.[7]

This was not purely a victory for philanthropic theories, since these alternatives often represented a cheaper form of provision, which made them acceptable to more economically minded authorities.

Nevertheless, the growing influence of the philanthropic approach can be seen in the increasing powers given to the Poor Law authorities to sever the links between children and their environments. Emigration was the most comprehensive way of achieving this objective but could be arranged for only comparatively few children. The next best alternative was the so-called "Poor Law adoption". The Poor Law Amendment Act 1889 provided that "where a child is maintained by the guardians of any [Poor Law] union and is deserted by its parent" or if the parent was "imprisoned as a result of an offence against the child", the guardians might resolve "that such child be under the control of the guardians until it reaches sixteen (if a boy) or eighteen (if a girl)". In 1899 this power was extended to include orphans and the children of parents who were "unfit". The result of such resolutions was to vest in the guardians all parental rights in the child in all matters except its religious upbringing. Although parents were given a right of appeal to a magistrates' court, the conferment on an administrative body of the power to assume legal control over children by its own executive act, unsupervised by any external body, was a dramatic extension of the state's authority over families, probably tolerated only because these were the families of the "disreputable" poor. These powers were inherited by local authority children's departments when they were created in 1948 and continued until the 1989 Act.

By the turn of the century, however, a new policy agenda was emerging as a result of concern over the implications for the national interest of the falling birth-rate and the physical degradation of the working class in a world of growing economic and military competitiveness. Considerable efforts were made through local authority public health and education departments to improve the basic health and sanitary conditions of all poor families. These remained administratively separate from the Poor Law, despite its absorption by the same authorities in the 1930s, but this new welfarist approach gradually undermined the policy of trying to remould the character of pauper children in isolation from their natural families. It was not until after the Second World War, though, that this change was reflected in legislation.

The 1948 reforms were brought about by the conjunction of a number of factors. As so often, the immediate trigger was a specific case. A thirteen-year-old boy (Dennis O'Neill) had died at the hands of his foster-parents while in the care of a local authority. Two inquiries, one by a prominent lawyer into the particular case and one by an interdepartmental committee into the general state of provision, revealed grossly inadequate standards of care and supervision for children in local authority care.[8] But the organizational changes recommended by these reports would not by themselves have led to the shift in policy towards working with families with a view to restoring children rather than seeking their permanent removal. This reflected the emphasis then being placed on the value of family life and the importance of the mother–child relationship as the post-war economy failed to integrate the large number of women who had been drawn into the labour force during the war. The newly created children's departments looked to the voluntary societies for their staff. By comparison with the Poor Law, the societies had been more concerned with the development of family casework and had strongly influenced such professional training as was available for social workers. All this suited the budgetary concerns of local authorities, who found the policy of rehabilitation cheaper than removal into institutional or foster care.

Even so, the Children Act 1948 went only part of the way towards the welfarist ideal. Its requirement that

the local authority shall, in all cases where it appears to them consistent with the welfare of the child so to do, endeavour to secure that the care of the child is taken over either (a) by a parent or guardian of his, or (b) by a relative or friend of his, being, where possible a person of the same religious persuasion[9]

said nothing about prevention. It was only in 1963 that children's departments acquired power to make provision in cash or kind to families for the purpose of reducing the need to take children into care.[10] But this power reflected the extent to which their focus had shifted away from deprived children, who had been the primary object of the former Poor Law, towards delinquents. Governments tend to be more willing to provide funds for the reduction of crime than the relief of distress.

Whatever its motives and limitations, the Children Act 1948 nevertheless embodied a significant piece of humanitarian rhetoric which marked a decisive break in the political perception of the community's duties towards children and, therefore, of its concept of children's rights. The public care of children was no longer to be focused on preparing them for service to the national economy. Instead, it became the duty of the authorities "to exercise their powers with respect to [the child] so as to further his best interests, and to afford him opportunity for the proper development of his character and abilities".[11]

By the late 1960s, the optimism which had underlain these rehabilitative and preventive goals had begun to fade. The problems of the national economy were simultaneously creating more work for the authorities while denying them a matching growth in resources. The ideals of rehabilitation appeared to be leading social workers[12] and judges[13] to put excessive value on a child's "blood ties", at the expense of his or her emotional relationships with foster-parents or prospective adopters. The consequent "tug-of-love" cases produced a good deal of adverse comment from the media and from some influential child care professionals. These problems led to the formation in 1969 of a Departmental Committee on the Adoption of Children (the Houghton Committee), which reported in 1972.[14]

The thrust of the recommendations of the Houghton Report was to strengthen the hands of local authorities in relation to the parents of children in their care. No child who had been in care for more than six months should be removed by a parent without twenty-eight days' notice; the power to assume parental rights by resolution should be exercisable simply on the fact that a child had been in care for three years or more; and a procedure should be introduced for the parents of a child in care to relinquish their child for adoption even though no prospective adopters had yet been found. The proposals received support from the publication in 1973 of a study, *Children Who Wait*, by Jane Rowe and Lydia Lambert.[15] This research, which had been commissioned by the Committee, indicated that many children were being denied permanent home placements while attempts, with very little hope of success, were made to solve the problems of their natural family. In these cases the rehabilitative goal was the enemy of clear planning for a child's future and simply resulted in vacillation and indecision.

The rapid introduction of legislation owes something to another notorious case, the death of Maria Colwell in 1973. Maria had been returned to her mother and step-father after spending five of her six years of life being fostered by her aunt. Shortly afterwards she was murdered by her step-father. An inquiry into the management of her care reported in 1974.[16] Although the Children Act 1975 was primarily concerned with implementing the major proposals of the Houghton Committee, which were largely irrelevant to this case, it also contained a number of new provisions as an immediate response to the Colwell report.

In the event, the Children Act 1975 was implemented only in a piecemeal fashion over the course of the following ten years. Whether as a result of the legislation itself or the policies with which it was associated, statistics show that, from the early 1970s, local authorities adopted a more conservative approach to the return of children in care to their families.[17] This shift in policy partly explains the impetus for the 1985 review. The disillusionment of the late 1960s and 1970s generated radically opposing critiques of child care law. Paradoxically, however, they converged on similar short-term reforms.

One view saw the failure of the rehabilitative and preventive policies of the 1960s as the result of insufficient commitment. It argued that inadequacies in child care could be prevented only by a radical redistribution of social resources and the elimination of inequality within society. On such a view the maintenance, even strengthening, of bureaucratic control over the children of the poor represented an extension of power by an authoritarian conservative state. It was a policy designed to remove the threat posed by poverty to the social order without eliminating its cause.

The other view drew on philosophies associated with the "new right". These argued that state restrictions on individual action were illegitimate exercises of power for which there was no moral basis. State intrusion into family life undermined the unique value which family autonomy provided in fostering a sense of individual responsibility. Expenditure on welfare services, then, could be justified, if at all, only for the most minimal functions. Similarly, it was taken as given that families knew better than state bureaucracies what was best for their members. The state could, therefore, never provide the range of response necessary to cater for the individual needs of children in care.

Holders of these perspectives found common cause in the issue of local authorities' discretion to control visits by parents to children in care. These powers were confirmed by the House of Lords in 1981[18] but, in 1983, statutory provisions were introduced which gave parents whose access was terminated, or to whom it had never been granted, the right to appeal against the decision to a magistrates' court.[19] Nevertheless, fundamental issues of the exercise of state power over families remained unresolved by this comparatively minor reform.

Child protection law

At the time of the 1985 Review, this area of law found its major expression in the Children and Young Persons Act 1969. Although now associated mainly with the problem of child abuse and neglect, its origins lie in the concern of Victorian England over the threat of disorder caused by the growth of delinquency associated with urban poverty. The development of reformatories as a constructive alternative to imprisonment for children who had committed offences was paralleled by the creation of industrial schools intended to give moral and vocational training to the class of children who were thought likely to become delinquents. In 1854 the courts were given a new power to send to those schools children (under fourteen) who had not committed any crime, but who were, for example, found begging or frequenting the company of reputed thieves, or who had been declared uncontrollable by their parents. The regimes of industrial schools and reformatories gradually became indistinguishable and it was thought to be accidental whether a child had come to official attention because he had committed an offence or because it was thought he might do so. In 1933 the two types of schools were legally assimilated and became known as "approved schools".

As the movement for reformatories and industrial schools gained increasing influence over the criminal justice system, many of its leaders turned their attention to the problem of protecting children from threats posed to them by their parents. This was not, however, so much a purely humane concern as a further extension of the attempt to prevent delinquency. Parental neglect or maltreatment of children was thought to make an important contribution to their development as criminals.

Of course the ordinary law of assault or homicide had always been used against parents whose ill-treatment of their children was so gross as to attract the attention of the prosecuting authorities. The English family has never been an entirely lawless zone, at least since reasonable records are available. But the criminal law could offer only limited protection. The Poor Law authorities were the first, in 1868, to acquire specific power to prosecute a parent who "wilfully neglected to provide adequate food, clothing, medical aid or lodging" for a child in his or her custody.[20] This, however, was primarily intended to reduce the financial burden on those authorities by giving them a means of pressuring parents who seemed to be too reliant on poor relief. It was only as a result of lobbying by the National Society for the Prevention of Cruelty to Children (established in 1889 through an amalgamation of local societies) that a general offence was created in 1889 in relation to *anyone* caring for a child who wilfully ill-treated, neglected or abandoned the child in a manner likely to cause unnecessary suffering or injury to health.[21] If a parent were convicted, the child could be committed to the charge of a relative or anyone else willing to have the child, and that person would acquire the rights of a parent over the child.

Of course, 1889 was also the year in which the Poor Law authorities acquired the power to pass resolutions assuming parental rights. This escalation of state interventionism has been linked[22] to the economic depression of the 1880s, which deepened concern about the disruptive effects of poverty and hastened the movement for moral reform of the poor. Those who failed to respond, in this case, by caring properly for their children, were to be punished. This created the conditions for the expansion of the child protection movement, although more positive concerns for the human stock of the nation were also beginning to emerge. Local authorities had, for instance, been given powers in 1872 to inspect premises in which children were being fostered for reward, and these were strengthened in 1897.[23]

The "National Efficiency" movement redefined problems of child welfare in the language of hygiene rather than of morality, although, in practice, it retained significant moral implications. The decline of an overtly "moral" basis for intervention had a very curious consequence, however. We have seen how, in 1933, "uncontrollable" children who were not delinquents, but might become so, were treated in a manner almost indistinguishable from children who had committed offences: they might be committed to an approved school ostensibly for their own good.[24] They were all children "in need of care and protection". But could it not equally be argued that children whose parents had injured them were also "in need of care and protection"? Moved by such considerations, these children were brought within the same legal category with the consequence that a court could commit them also to an approved school.[25] While it was nobody's intention that maltreated children should actually be managed in the same way as delinquents or near-delinquents, this assimilation shows how official perceptions of their distinctiveness as a group had faded.

From the 1930s until the 1970s, the attention of policy-makers was almost exclusively directed at the problem of delinquency. Children "in need of care and protection" were thought to be actual or potential delinquents, and the legislation which was to become the Children and Young Persons Act 1969 and which provided the only procedure for dealing with cases of child abuse and neglect was mainly designed to deal with child offenders. By seeing delinquency as a product of deprivation, neglect, in its turn, became indistinguishable from delinquency. The result was that, under the structure of the 1969 Act, the local authority "brought the child" before the court, whether "the child" was a teenage vandal or a battered baby; parents were not true parties to the case; the usual disposition was an order committing the child into care or requiring the child to submit to supervision; and only the child could bring an appeal, which went to the Crown Court, the major criminal court in England and Wales.

The Maria Colwell inquiry in 1974 did much to re-awaken concern about child abuse. But a single incident would not on its own have been sufficient to bring about the surge of activity which took place during the 1970s. The movement had started in the USA in the 1960s in the field of paediatric medicine where Dr Henry Kempe and his colleagues in Denver claimed to have identified the "battered baby syndrome". Their campaign attracted a good deal of support within the medical profession because it represented a new challenge in a field which had overcome most of the major causes of infant mortality. This does not, however, explain the public enthusiasm for the issue. To understand this, we must remember that, following the assassination of President Kennedy in 1963, the 1960s were notorious for the degree of self-scrutiny to which American society subjected itself. Radical concerns for civil rights, poverty and, later, the injustices of the war in Vietnam were matched by conservative anxieties about drug abuse, sexual promiscuity, the increasing instability of marriage and the family and, of course, crime. Child abuse could be identified as an explanatory factor by each group. The conservatives restated the nineteenth-century view that "defective" personalities were created in individuals who experienced violence from their parents. The violent society could be explained by the moral failure of that most cherished institution, the family. Extreme measures could be justified to reclaim families and to protect society. But a competing radical thesis saw child abuse as a consequence of a society riven by inequality, injustice and institutionalized violence. The phenomenon could then become the basis for a crusade to restructure that society.

There is little doubt that these ideological factors also played a large part in the spread of interest in child abuse and neglect in the United Kingdom during the 1970s. The response was a series of administrative measures taken within the Department of Health and Social Security for managing child abuse and neglect cases, including the establishment of Area Review Committees, At-Risk Registers and the use of case conferences. Coupled with the more cautious attitudes of social services departments about returning children once they had come into care, these developments were increasingly criticized during the late 1970s and early 1980s. Pressure groups, such as the Family Rights Group, Justice for Children and the Children's Legal Centre, were formed in the belief that welfare authorities were paying too little regard to the rehabilitative and preventive goals of the post-war years. As controls upon public expenditure tightened, further restricting the attainability of those goals, the portrayal of child protection practice as a growing form of class oppression seemed increasingly plausible. However, the rate at which children *actually came into care* during the 1970s in fact *decreased*, although, as we have seen, when they were in care, they tended to stay for longer periods.[26] The numbers of children removed under the emergency powers of place of safety orders did increase during this period, which seems to indicate a greater readiness to take immediate formal action in cases of suspected abuse and neglect. But the fall in the number of committals to care shows that the vast number of these orders did not lead to extended removal of children from parental care. Although this might be interpreted as an indication that the original order was inappropriate, it could also be seen as a sign that the authorities were more willing to seek a non-compulsory outcome, despite proper initial concerns.

The Social Services Committee also advised caution in the evaluation of statistical trends in the numbers of children in care and warned against uncritical attempts simply to reduce the number. Nevertheless, it acknowledged the existence of a widespread view "that there are too many children in care".[27] Quite apart from these questions, the attempt to force child protection law into a framework designed for juvenile offenders had produced so many anomalies and deficiencies that a thorough review was felt to be essential.

The wardship jurisdiction

Historically, this is the oldest part of the legal machinery which could be mobilized to establish legal controls over children's welfare. It developed in medieval times to regulate the inheritance of landed wealth. Wardship was the right to look after land inherited by a child whose father had died before the child had come of age. This could be a valuable right because the guardian was entitled to the profits from the land and might also be able to arrange a marriage for the child that would advance his own interests. Disputes about the choice of guardian or the exercise of his responsibilities came before the King's courts. But their primary interest was in the child's property rather than his or her personal welfare. This was equally the case where the court controlled decisions about the ward's marriage. The preoccupation with property led to the practice that the wardship jurisdiction would be exercised only where the ward had property to protect. However, the rule could be substantially evaded by settling a token sum of money on the child before applying for wardship. In 1949 even this nominal linkage with the historical origins of the jurisdiction was broken, when anyone who could claim a legitimate interest in the child was permitted to institute wardship proceedings.

Modern wardship procedure has two important aspects. One is the relative informality of the procedure and the potential speed at which it can be activated. The child becomes a ward immediately the application is made but will cease to be one unless an appointment is made within twenty-one days to hear the case. The appointment will be dealt with by a registrar, who has limited powers, but the hearing itself must be before a High Court (or Deputy High Court) judge. Much of the argument is submitted in writing, although this may be supplemented by oral evidence. The judge has the utmost freedom in assessing this as the normal rules about the admissibility of evidence do not apply.

The second feature is that, having formed a view of the child's best interests, the judge has extremely wide powers to take whatever measures he or she deems appropriate in the child's interests. The judge may, for example, forbid,[28] or authorize,[29] the sterilization of the child, override parental objections to a life-saving operation,[30] and forbid references to the identity of a child or the parents in the press.[31] No important step in the life of a ward may be made without the permission of the court.

The number of wardship applications rose sharply in the 1970s, from just 622 in 1971 to 2,815 in 1985. This seems to have been due to an increasing readiness by local authorities to use this procedure to obtain control over a child where other child welfare law would not permit. But there were also disadvantages in this course of action. Wardship proceedings are expensive, since they require the employment of counsel. Although they can be quickly started, they can take a very long time to be completed, especially if the court appoints the Official Solicitor to represent the child. Furthermore, even if the child is eventually committed into local authority care, he or she remains a ward and the social services department's actions are subject to the court's supervision. On the other hand, the pressures building up during the late 1970s against the use of state power might have pushed some local authorities towards wardship. It is possible that the structural weaknesses of care proceedings lessened their value to the authorities as a means of achieving the protection (as they saw it) of children.

Many of the reported cases from the wardship jurisdiction over this period show that it was also used by parents and others in attempts to challenge the local authorities' exercise of their discretionary powers. In 1981 the House of Lords tried to check this development by ruling that, where a local authority possessed powers under child welfare law to make decisions concerning a particular child, the High Court should not attempt to deal with these matters. The only circumstances where it might intervene were where it could be shown that the authority had made some serious error or acted very unreasonably.[32] This ruling did not seem to settle the matter, and in 1985 the House of Lords reaffirmed it in even stronger terms. It was not just a question of practice, the court asserted; the child welfare law statutes (such as the Children and Young Persons Act 1969 and the Child Care Act 1980) actually prohibited the use of the wardship jurisdiction for such purposes.[33]

In 1987 the Law Commission examined the wardship jurisdiction and expressed concern about its relationship to other areas of child welfare law, which were governed by precisely worded statutes. This was accentuated by the fear that the consensus over reforms in the statutory codes which had been established by the Child Care Law Review could simply be bypassed by the use of the wardship jurisdiction.[34] One solution considered was the abolition of wardship and the incorporation of some of its aspects into the new legislation. However, many people, especially the judges of the High Court, felt that the jurisdiction was a useful safety net to deal with unexpected and difficult situations for which the statutory procedures might prove too inflexible. This argument received a boost when the wardship jurisdiction was used to review many of the cases of children alleged to be victims of sexual abuse in Cleveland. The problem was of reconciling the retention of the wardship jurisdiction for difficult cases, while preventing it from displacing the statutory system, constructed by Parliament. We shall see in Chapter 3 how this has been tackled in the 1989 Act.

One feature of the wardship jurisdiction could, however, prove fatal in due course. The European Convention on Human Rights and Fundamental Freedoms, to which the United Kingdom is a signatory, stipulates, in Article 6, that "in the determination of his civil rights and obligations ... everyone is entitled to a fair and public hearing within a reasonable time by an independent and impartial tribunal established by law." The European Court of Human Rights has decided that a parent's right to visit his or her child is a civil right to which the Convention refers[35] and so too, presumably, is the right of parents to bring up their own children. Yet, in exercising the wardship jurisdiction, judges must base their decisions only on their view of the child's interests. It is by no means clear that the "rights" of parents play any part in this decision. If that is so, wardship may well contravene the Convention.

The divorce jurisdiction

In 1950, as an experiment, a "court welfare officer" was appointed to the Divorce Division of the High Court in London to investigate and report, when requested by the court, on the circumstances of children in divorce proceedings. He was later assisted by officers from the probation service, which also began to provide similar help in cases which arose outside the capital. These developments received statutory recognition in the Matrimonial Proceedings (Children) Act 1958.

The divorce courts have made extensive use of the power to order welfare reports when they have had to decide which of two disputing parents should be awarded custody of their children. Such disputes probably occur in less than 10 per cent of divorce cases in which children are involved.[36] Nevertheless, the 1958 Act required that in no case should a divorce decree be made absolute (fully effective) unless the judge accepted that the arrangements made for the children were satisfactory or the best that could be devised in the circumstances.

It proved difficult to establish a means by which judges could satisfy themselves that proper arrangements were being made for children by divorcing parents, especially if the parents were not in dispute about this. A judge could order parents to produce further information by means of an affidavit (sworn statement) and also instruct a welfare officer to investigate the children's circumstances. In exceptional cases the judge could order continued supervision of the children by the welfare officer or local authority social services or even commit them to the care of the local authority. It appeared that judges asked for further information of some kind in about 10 per cent of cases, especially if many children were involved, if they were divided between the parents or if the father was going to look after them.[37] But Care or Supervision Orders were rarely made.

The problem of ensuring that proper arrangements had been made for the children became more difficult when, in 1977, the rules were altered to allow a court to grant a divorce without either of the parties attending a hearing. In an attempt to sustain the court's supervisory role where children were involved, the new rules required the person who filed the divorce petition (usually the wife) to complete a form stating what arrangements were proposed for the children and attend an appointment with the judge. Research published in 1983 showed that these appointments were conducted with varying degrees of formality.[38] Most were so perfunctory that it was unlikely that they were very effective. In 1985 a Committee appointed to review matrimonial procedures recommended that attempts should be made to reinforce this process by requiring more detailed information to be presented to the judge[39] and in 1986 the Law Commission appeared to agree.[40] In 1987 the Law Commission examined the use of Supervision Orders made in divorce cases and suggested various improvements.[41]

Some of these procedures have been changed by the 1989 Act. But the Act also introduces more fundamental reforms in the concepts which underlie orders controlling where children should live after divorce and their relationships with their parents, following the Law Commission's recommendations in its 1986 Review of Child Custody Law.[42] The words "custody" and "access" disappear completely. However, the 1989 Act still does not fully resolve the basic issues as to the extent and manner of court attempts to supervise the interests of children caught up in divorce, if indeed this should be done at all.

Notes

1. *Second Report from the Social Services Committee* (HC 360), London: HMSO, March 1984, vol. 1, para. 119.
2. DHSS, *Review of Child Care Law: Report to Ministers of an Interdepartmental Working Party*, London: HMSO, 1985; *The Law on Child Care and Family Services*, Cm 62, London: HMSO, 1987.
3. See Law Commission, *Eighteenth Annual Report 1982–3*, Law Com. No. 131, London: HMSO, 1984, para. 2.43.
4. Law Commission, *Family Law: Review of Child Law: Guardianship and Custody*, Law Com. No. 172, London: HMSO, 1988; Law Commission, *Family Law: Review of Child Law: Wards of Court*, Working Paper No. 101, London: HMSO, 1987.
5. *A Child in Trust: The Report of the Panel of Inquiry into the circumstances surrounding the Death of Jasmine Beckford*, London Borough of Brent, 1985; *Report of the Inquiry into Child Abuse in Cleveland 1987*, Cm. 412, London: HMSO, 1988; *Whose Child? The Report of the Public Inquiry into the Death of Tyra Henry*, London Borough of Lambeth, 1987; *A Child in Mind: Report of the Commission of Inquiry into the circumstances surrounding the Death of Kimberley Carlile*, London Borough of Greenwich, 1987.
6. *Commentaries on the Laws of England* 1.16.1.
7. Jean Heywood, *Children in Care*, London: Routledge & Kegan Paul, 1978, p. 90.
8. *Report by Sir Walter Monckton on the circumstances which led to the*

boarding-out of Dennis and Terence O'Neill, Cmd 6636, London: HMSO, 1945; *Report of the Care of Children (Curtis) Committee*, Cmd 6922, London: HMSO, 1946.

9. Children Act 1948, s. 1(3).
10. Children and Young Persons Act 1963, s. 1; later Child Care Act 1980, s. 1.
11. Children Act 1948, s. 12(1); later, Child Care Act 1980, s. 18.
12. See Nigel Parton, *The Politics of Child Abuse*, London: Macmillan, 1985, pp. 89–90.
13. A leading case, given much contemporary publicity, was *re C. (M.A.) (An Infant)* [1966] 1 WLR 646; see the discussion of this and other cases by Naomi Michaels, "The Dangers of a Change of Parentage in Custody and Adoption Cases" (1967) 83 *Law Quarterly Review* 547–68.
14. *Report of the Departmental Committee on the Adoption of Children*, Cmnd 5107, London: HMSO, 1972.
15. Jane Rowe and Lydia Lambert, *Children who Wait*, London: Association of British Adoption Agencies, 1973.
16. *Report of the Committee of Inquiry into the Care and Supervision provided in relation to Maria Colwell*, London: HMSO, 1974.
17. Robert Dingwall and John Eekelaar, "Rethinking Child Protection", in M.D.A. Freeman (ed.) *State, Law and the Family: Critical Perspectives*, London: Tavistock, 1984; Parton, *op.cit.*, p. 124.
18. *A. v. Liverpool City Council* [1982] AC 363.
19. Health and Social Services and Social Security Adjudications Act 1983, s. 6.
20. Poor Law Amendment Act 1868, s. 37; see now Children and Young Persons Act 1933, s. 1.
21. Prevention of Cruelty to and Protection of Children Act 1889, s. 1.
22. Parton, *op.cit.*, p. 32.
23. Infant Life Protection Acts 1862–97.
24. Children and Young Persons Act 1933.
25. Children and Young Persons Act 1933.
26. Dingwall and Eekelaar, *op.cit.;* Parton, *op.cit.*, p. 124.
27. *Select Committee Report*, vol. 1, para. 20.
28. *re D. (A Minor) (Wardship: Sterilisation)* [1976] Fam 185.
29. *re B. (A Minor) (Wardship: Sterilisation)* [1987] 2 WLR 1213.
30. *re B. (A Minor) (Wardship: Medical Treatment)* [1981] 1 WLR 1421.
31. *X County Council v. A.* [1984] 1 WLR 1422.
32. *A. v. Liverpool City Council* [1982] AC 363.
33. *re W.* [1985] AC 791.
34. Law Commission, *Wards of Court*, Working Paper No. 101, London: HMSO, 1987.
35. *R. v. United Kingdom and other cases*, Judgments and Decisions of the European Court of Human Rights, vol. 120 and vol. 121 (July 1987).
36. John Eekelaar and Eric Clive, *Custody after Divorce*, Oxford: SSRC Centre for Socio-Legal Studies, 1977.
37. See note 21.
38. G. Davis, A. MacLeod and M. Murch, "Undefended Divorces: Should

Section 41 of the Matrimonial Causes Act be Repealed?" (1983) 46 *Modern Law Review* 121.

39. *Report of the Matrimonial Causes Procedure Committee (Booth Committee)*, London: HMSO, 1985.
40. Law Commission, *Review of Child Law: Custody*, Working Paper No. 96, London: HMSO, 1986.
41. Law Commission, *Care, Supervision and Interim Orders in Custody Proceedings*, Working Paper No. 100, London: HMSO, 1987.
42. See note 40.

Chapter two

A new framework for private law: parental responsibility and children's rights

The 1989 Act is an attempt to take a fresh look at the balance struck between the interests of parents, children and the wider community. Most of it is concerned with the conditions under which the *state* should intervene in the relationship between parents and their children, and therefore concerns *public* law. However, the Select Committee, the Working Party, the Law Commission and, eventually, the Government also reviewed the legal relationship between children and their parents. Over the years, the uncoordinated development of legislation and its interpretation by the courts had created a hodgepodge of rights, powers and duties and a confusing array of court orders. Since these control the distribution of rights which individual adults may have in relation to children and do not necessarily involve the state, they are usually referred to as *private* law. While most of this book is devoted to the public law of child care, this chapter focuses on the changes made to private law by the 1989 Act.

Parental responsibility and parents' rights

The law usually employs the concept of "rights" to determine people's legal entitlements in relation to each other and towards certain objects. However, no Act of Parliament has ever clearly established *what* rights parents have regarding their children, or even that they have any such rights at all. What are we to make of a provision which says

> In this Act, unless the context otherwise requires, "the parental rights and duties" means as respects a particular child (whether legitimate or not), all the rights and duties which by law the

mother and father have in relation to a legitimate child and his property.

[*Children Act 1975, s. 85(1)*]

Or,

In relation to the custody or upbringing of a minor, and in relation to the administration of any property belonging to or held in trust for a minor or the application of income of any such property, a mother shall have the same rights and authority as the law allows to a father, and the rights and authority of mother and father shall be equal and exercisable by either without the other.

[*Guardianship Act 1973, s. 1(1)*]

But *what* rights does a mother or father have "by law"; what *are* the "rights and authority" which the law allows? Neither of those Acts, both of which were repealed by the 1989 Act, gave any answer.

The new Act tries to develop a different approach based on the concept of "parental responsibility". It proclaims:

Where a child's father and mother were married to each other at the time of his birth, they shall each have parental responsibility for the child.

[*s. 2(1)*]

And

... "parental responsibility" means all the rights, duties, powers, responsibilities and authority which by law a parent of a child has in relation to the child and his property.

[*s. 3(1)*]

But this no more answers the question: "*what* rights does a parent have?" than did the repealed provisions.

Nevertheless, although the "rights" of parents have never been laid down systematically, it is clear that the law makes much the same assumptions as ordinary people. A hospital would be acting unlawfully if it handed a baby over to anyone other than the parents, unless it had special legal authority to do otherwise. So parents have a right to possess their child;[1] they can give the child any name they choose;[2] they can consent to a child's being given medical treatment, even though the child may object (but see p. 24), send the child to a school of their choice and even administer "reasonable chastisement".

But these are really better understood as parental *privileges* rather than parental *rights*. They are limited both by the possibility of legal review and by the extent to which children may be thought to have competing claims. It is, however, striking that the 1989 Act prefers to bracket all these privileges under the general expression "responsibility". When we go on to discover how tenaciously the new Act fixes parents (at least, certain parents) with this "responsibility", we may begin to suspect that this choice of phrasing reflects a more sectarian ideological commitment than the broad bipartisan support for the 1989 Act might imply. It certainly needs to be seen in the context of the general Conservative belief in the desirability of privatizing the responsibility for the care of dependent individuals, including children, and the diminution of any role for the state.

Who has "parental responsibility" and how is it lost?

The general rule about parental responsibility being held by each parent, if married to each other, is set out in *section 2(1)*, which we have just quoted. The same principle applies if the child's father marries the mother after the child's birth [*s. 2(3)*]. But if the parents were not married to each other, the law gives responsibility exclusively to the mother [*s. 2(2)*]. Even if the father lives with the mother, his opinions and wishes have no legal relevance.

Under the old law, the father could achieve equal parental rights only by marrying the mother or adopting the child jointly with her. He could have applied for "custody" under the Guardianship of Minors Act 1971, but that was an all-or-nothing procedure: either he obtained all "rights" in the child (they could not be shared) or failed completely. This was modified by the Family Law Reform Act 1987 which allowed a father to apply to a court for an order giving him some "parental rights and duties", which could be shared. The 1989 Act now allows an unmarried father to apply to a court for an order giving him "parental responsibility" for his child [*s. 4(1) (a)*]. But this might be a costly and cumbersome procedure. So the Act also allows unmarried parents to *make an agreement* that the father may share parental responsibility with the mother [*s. 4(1) (b)*]. This agreement (which the Act calls "a parental responsibility agreement") must be "recorded", in a manner to be specified by regulations, probably in court, so there will still be a degree of formality, but the procedure is intended to be simple. If a father has obtained parental responsibility in any one of these ways, his legal position becomes the same as that of a married father with respect to his children.

How may a parent lose this responsibility? Of course, if a parent dies, parental responsibility can pass to a guardian, who may either be appointed by the parent during his or her lifetime or, after the parent's death, by a court [s. 5 and s. 6]. But, while a mother, or the father who is married to her, remains alive, they cannot surrender their responsibility to anyone else [s. 2(9)] except through the mechanism of adoption (which has been little affected by the 1989 Act and is not dealt with in this book). They may arrange for some or all of their responsibilities to be met by others on their behalf, and some court orders made under the 1989 Act may control their exercise of their responsibility. But the ultimate responsibility for the child remains on their shoulders. In the case of the unmarried father who obtained parental responsibility by court order or under a "parental responsibility agreement" the position is different. This man may lose his responsibility by court order if this is sought by anyone else with such responsibility (say, the mother) or the child [s. 4(3)]. But the child's mother (if alive) will keep her responsibility. Under the Act, there is no way in which parental responsibility acquired on a child's birth by the mother or a married father can be passed over to the state. This is a change of profound importance, the ramifications of which will be explored in Chapters 3 and 10.

Shared parental responsibility

It is an important principle of the Act that a person does not lose parental responsibility just because someone else acquires it [s. 2(6)] unless this is specifically provided for by law, as in the case of adoption. So parental responsibility can be shared. Normally this will be between the parents as described above, although other people may acquire parental responsibility, notably under a Residence Order (see p. 26) or a Care Order (dealt with in Chapters 7 and 10). Parents may, therefore, find themselves sharing parental responsibility with people who are not the child's parents.

Where parental responsibility is shared, the Act provides that anybody who holds it can make decisions about a child on their own, without consulting the other party or parties, except where the Act specifically requires joint consent [*s. 2(7)*]. So, if a child is living with a person with parental responsibility, that person can make decisions which necessarily arise from caring for the child. But if anybody else has an interest in the child, their opinions will have equal weight. It is hoped that people with parental responsibility will normally act in agreement with each other. If they cannot agree, the Act provides for the dispute to be resolved by a court through a Specific Issue Order or a Prohibited Steps Order (see p. 27–8). The burden for seeking the order lies on the person who wants to *prevent* a particular course of action being taken by another who has parental responsibility.

Children's rights

None of the official documents leading up to the 1989 Act had much to say about children's rights, although this was actually a very important issue among the groups of academics, practitioners and lobbyists seeking reform. The concept of "children's rights" was used in two ways. First, it referred to a general aspiration to improve the conditions of children not just in this country but throughout the world. This sense is reflected in the movement for an international convention on children's rights whose catalogue of entitlements is essentially a political programme expressing certain ideals of social justice. The second, and narrower, interpretation of the concept refers to the extent to which children are recognized as having some degree of personal autonomy. How far can a child resist a course of action that an adult (usually a parent) wishes to impose and determine for him or herself what should happen?[3] If a child is not legally considered to be an adult until the age of eighteen, can a parent compel a seventeen-year-old to undergo medical treatment to which the child objects because the parent thinks this is good for the child (and even if it *is* actually good for him or her)? Could it mean that the parent could *prevent* treatment being given if the parent thinks (correctly or not) that it would *not* be good for the child?

The 1989 Act virtually ignores these questions. As we shall see, it does specify that, in certain contexts, courts or welfare authorities must give particular attention to the wishes and feelings of the children with whom they are dealing and special provisions have been enacted permitting children in some circumstances to refuse to undergo medical examination. But, apart from that, it seems that the decision-maker's views will normally take priority over those of the child if there is a disagreement. The Act has nothing to say about what happens when an ordinary person with parental responsibility has a difference of opinion with the child as to how that responsibility ought to be exercised. These are sensitive questions and the other important reforms introduced by the Act might have been delayed by the controversy if they had been tackled. But the law has already had to confront some of them and the courts' decisions are important constraints on the way the Act can be used.

Existing legislation already gives children of sixteen and over the clear right to decide for themselves about whether or not to seek or accept medical treatment.[4] They do not need parental consent, nor can parents force treatment on them. But what if the child is under sixteen? The House of Lords held in the *Gillick* case that a girl under sixteen *could* consent to contraceptive treatment without obtaining the approval of her parents, provided she was sufficiently mature, both intellectually and emotionally, to understand its nature and implications.[5] As a result of this decision it seems that, provided the "maturity test" is satisfied, parents can neither compel nor prevent medical treatment. This would not, for example, hold up the vaccination of a baby, because the infant would be unable to weigh the risks and benefits for him or herself. But it would mean that a fourteen-year-old boy could decline minor cosmetic surgery for the improvement of a hare-lip repaired in infancy, even if his parents wanted the operation to be performed.

It has been argued that the "maturity" test implies that the child's wishes should be respected only if the doctor thinks the child is acting in his or her own best interests.[6] On a strict reading of the *Gillick* decision, we think this interpretation is wrong.[7] It would be strange if the child's capacity to make a decision depended on some third party's assessment of his or her best interests. This would undermine the central theme of the decision, which was to assert the independent legal capacity of a child who satisfied the "maturity test". It will be seen that the 1989 Act adopts this approach on the occasions when it specifies that a "mature" child can resist medical or psychiatric assessment or examination even, presumably, where the refusal is against his or her interests (see pp. 86, 91, 135).

It would be rash to believe that the *Gillick* judgment is the last word on the matter. The courts are clearly grappling with decisions about where to draw the line across which the generations negotiate with each other. In that case Lord Scarman framed his judgment in very general terms. Suppose that parents object to a fifteen-year-old's attending the ceremonies of a religious sect of which they disapprove. Could they seek an injunction against the sect forbidding them from contacting the child, and should it be granted if the court believes the child is acting against his or her interests? At perhaps the most extreme, can a child of sufficient maturity leave home and live with someone else, even if their parents object? *Section 20(11)* allows a child of sixteen to live in local authority accommodation against the parents' wishes. If the courts concede the basic principle that a mature child has the right to make such decisions, they may modify it by ruling that children who make choices which are obviously detrimental to their welfare must, by definition, lack the maturity to benefit from the principle. This would preserve considerable opportunities for the imposition of adult values on children.

The question of punishment raises a special problem. The Education Act 1986 forbids the corporal punishment of children who are receiving state-funded education. But where does this leave parents who beat their children, or in other ways restrict their liberty? The law has always allowed parents the privilege of "reasonable chastisement". But does the *Gillick* principle allow a parent to inflict physical punishment or restraint upon a mature child who objects to it? It is at least arguable that parents have lost their legal protection from a charge of criminal assault in such circumstances. Some have argued that we should follow the examples of Sweden, Denmark, Finland and Norway and pass laws declaring that any form of child-beating is unlawful. This would indicate social disapproval of a culture which tolerates a certain measure of violence towards children and treats child abuse merely as an extreme form of otherwise acceptable behaviour, giving it a certain legitimacy and creating difficulties for courts and welfare agencies in setting and enforcing standards.[8] "Excessive" punishment by a parent might constitute grounds for bringing care proceedings, as discussed in Chapter 7.

The development of case law on the degree of autonomy which should be afforded to children must necessarily influence the use of the 1989 Act in two ways. First, those agencies which may acquire parental responsibility need to be very sensitive to the extent to which that power is used to impose decisions on a child and to the weight they should give to the child's views as against those of natural parents. We have referred to some express provisions concerning medical or psychiatric assessment. But it is also probably unlawful for a local authority to prevent a mature girl in their care from seeking contraception, even if her parents or, indeed, councillors object on moral grounds. Second, these decisions may provide the basis for a widening of the circumstances when an authority may become involved on the initiative of a mature child against parental decisions. It is not difficult, for example, to envisage an occasion on which a mature child from a South Asian family rejected a parental decision to return to the home country and sought help in resisting this.

A new range of orders

When married parents separate or divorce, it is often necessary to make decisions about how their responsibilities for a child are to be distributed between them. Under the old laws, the court would, usually, make a custody order in favour of one parent (normally the mother) and an access order in favour of the other. Sometimes a "joint" custody order was made. Unfortunately, there was considerable confusion about what the expression "custody" really meant. The position of parents who had *not* been granted custody was particularly unclear: did they have a right, for example, to be consulted over questions such as the child's schooling or religious upbringing?[9]

With the new concept of "parental responsibility", it became necessary to re-structure the types of orders a court can make. The new law therefore does away with the concept of "custody" altogether. If the child is a child of both the parents, then, since they will have been married to each other, each will have equal parental responsibility (see p. 21). The court can now make a variety of orders, which are likely to become known as "Section 8 Orders" after their location in the Act. These do not deprive either parent of their ultimate responsibility for the child, but are intended to settle certain practical aspects of the exercise of that responsibility between the parents and provide a means of resolving disputes should they occur.

A *Residence Order* sets out the arrangements to be made as to the person with whom the child is to live; a *Contact Order* may require the person with whom the child lives to allow the child to visit or receive visits from another person or maintain contact with that person in other ways (e.g. by letter or telephone); a *Prohibited Steps Order* can state a specified aspect of parental responsibility (e.g.

taking the child abroad) cannot be exercised without the court's permission; a *Specific Issue Order* can give positive directions as to how any aspect of parental responsibility should be exercised [*s. 8*]. The Law Commission thought that courts should be discouraged from making orders as a matter of routine, so the court must not make an order unless it thinks that to do this would be better for the child than making no order at all [*s. 1(5)*].

Although these orders will be normally be made only in divorce proceedings, it is important to be aware that they can also be made in other family proceedings, including the new-style care proceedings under the 1989 Act. Residence and Contact Orders cannot be made in favour of a local authority [*s. 9(2)*] but such orders can be made in care proceedings (which we shall discuss in Chapter 7) to people who could apply for them in divorce cases. Residence Orders may become an important channel through which children leave compulsory care.

Section 8 Orders cannot be made after a child reaches sixteen unless the court thinks the circumstances are exceptional [*s. 9(7)*]. So, in the normal course, they will lapse when the child reaches that age [*s. 91(10)*] and courts should not make them extend beyond the child's sixteenth birthday unless the circumstances are exceptional [*s. 9(6)*].

Who can apply for an order?

Any parent, or guardian of a child and any person who has a Residence Order with respect to a child can apply for *any* of these new orders [*s. 10(4)*], either within divorce proceedings, other family proceedings or as a separate matter [*s. 10(1) (a)*]. *Any other person* (including the child) may ask the court for *permission* to apply for *any* of the orders [*s. 10(2) (b)*]. In deciding whether to give permission, the court has to take into account the applicant's connection with the child, the risk of the application disrupting the child's life and (if the child is being looked after by a local authority) that authority's plans and the views of the child's parents [*s. 10(9)*]. It should be noticed that an unmarried father is a "parent", even if he does not automatically have parental responsibility, and that he has a right, therefore, to apply for any of the Section 8 Orders. If a Residence Order is made in his favour, then the court must at the same time make an order giving him parental responsibility (if he does not already have it) because it would be wrong for him to be looking after the child without it [*s. 12(1)*].

Certain categories of people may apply for *Residence* or *Contact Orders* (but not the other orders) *without first obtaining permission*. They are:

1 Where the adults are not *both* the parents of the child in question, an adult who is not a parent of the child but who has treated the child as if the child were a member of the family during a marriage;

2 A person with whom the child has been living for at least three years (this need not be a continuous period, but must have begun within five years, and not have ended more than three months, before the application was made);

3 Any other person, if all persons who have parental responsibility for the child or who have a residence order in their favour with respect to a child, consent; or if the child is in care, if the local authority consents [*s. 10(5)*];

4 (Anyone who has obtained a Section 8 Order or who is named in a Contact Order can apply for its variation or discharge [*s. 10(6)*]).

The purpose is to make it easy for certain people, besides the child's parents or those with a Residence Order, who have a real interest in a child to have their "claim" to look after or keep contact with the child heard. These people may include step-parents [category (1) in the above list], foster-parents (perhaps relatives) who have long been caring for a child under a private arrangement [category (2)], local authority foster-parents [categories (2) and (3)] and indeed anyone else if the people who currently have parental responsibility agree to the application [category (3)]. It should be noted that although foster-parents have a *right* to apply for a Residence or Contact Order if they fall within category (2), they cannot exercise it without the consent of the local authority if the child has been with them for less than three years and they are not related to the child [*s. 9(3)*] (see p. 145).

Finally, the court can make any of these Section 8 Orders on its own initiative if it believes that it would be in the child's interests [*s. 10(1) (b)*].

There are some exceptions to this scheme. Residence and Contact Orders cannot be made in favour of local authorities; and if a child is in care (the new concept of care created by the 1989 Act will be explained in Chapter 5), the *only* Section 8 Order *anyone* (even a parent) can seek with respect to the child is a Residence Order [*s. 9(1) & (2)*]. These points will be considered in Chapter 10.

The effect of Residence Orders

When parents divorce or separate, it is usually necessary to decide which parent will keep the children. By discarding the concept of "custody" and concentrating on the practicalities, the Law Commission hoped that some of the tensions would be removed from such decisions. A Residence Order will just state the living arrangements and will say nothing about parental responsibility, which will continue to be shared. But it may contain detailed directions and impose conditions on parents and other people living with the child [*s. 11(7)*] and these may be enforced by monetary penalties imposed by magistrates [*s. 14(1)*]. The Act expressly envisages that a child may live with more than one person [*s. 11(4)*]. So a court might say that a child should live with one parent during school term and the other during the holidays.

If a court makes a Residence Order for a child to live with someone who is not a parent or guardian, and who would not otherwise have parental responsibility, the Act states that that person "shall have parental responsibility for the child while the residence order remains in force" [*s. 12(2)*]. The objective is to provide a way of recognizing the relationship between children and those adults with whom they are living in situations short of full adoption. This was previously attempted by the clumsy device of "custodianship orders" under the Children Act 1975 or Custody Orders under the matrimonial legislation. As we remarked earlier, if a Residence Order is made in favour of a father who does not have parental responsibility (e.g. if he is not married to the child's mother) then the court *must* also make an order giving him that responsibility [*s. 12(1)*] which he will retain even if the child later goes to live with someone else.

The consequence of Residence Orders is that parental responsibility is *shared* between the parents (or whoever had the responsibility before the order) and the new person or persons named in the order. As we have seen, sharing parental responsibility does not require consultation; irresolvable differences will have to be decided by a Specific Issue Order (see p. 23). If the person with the Residence

Order is *not* a parent of the child, though, the Act specifically states that he or she cannot arrange for the child's adoption or appoint a guardian [*s. 12(3)*]; nor give the child a new surname, nor take the child out of the United Kingdom for more than one month without the the written consent of everyone who has parental responsibility (or the permission of the court, which can be granted in advance when the Residence Order is made) [*s. 13*].

Practitioners will need to invent a word to describe a person who is caring for a child under a Residence Order. Such a person, if not already a parent, has somewhat fewer powers than a parent or legally appointed guardian. We think "residential guardian" might be an appropriate term.

The basis of the courts' decisions

Under the law in operation before the 1989 Act, when a child's parents were disputing with each other or with a local authority about where the child should live or what contact he or she should have with a separated parent, the courts always had to decide the matter on the basis that the child's welfare was the "first and paramount consideration". The Law Commission wanted to do away with this stylized expression and to say that:

> When determining any question under this Act the welfare of the child shall be the court's only concern.[10]

However, *section 1(1)* has retained the old formulation:

> When a court determines any question with respect to
>
> (a)   the upbringing of a child; or
>
> (b)   the administration of a child's property or the application of any income arising from it, the child's welfare shall be the court's *paramount* consideration.
>
> (emphasis added)

Unfortunately it has become unclear what the word "paramount" means. For some people, it means, in effect, the only consideration because the child's welfare rules over all other matters.[11] But this has been challenged by the view that the word simply means that a judge should give the child's interest special consideration in balancing it against other claims.[12]

The Act's preference for the traditional words may reflect some unease that the Law Commission's suggestion could make the duty to promote the child's welfare too absolute. Since it is sometimes uncertain *which* decision is best for a child, judges can be strongly tempted to allow the claims of other people to tip the balance. Although there may be some occasions when the immediate welfare of a child might arguably need to be sacrificed for the greater good of all children (such as returning a child kidnapped by one parent so as to discourage kidnapping)[13] it seems to us better that arguments over children should be framed in language directed at securing the interests of the child in question. If this is not done the result may be that those interests are entirely forgotten.

The new legislation does, however, try to clarify what judges should consider. For example, it is expressly stated that "the court shall have regard to the general principle that any delay in determining the question is likely to prejudice the welfare of the child" [*s. 1(2)*]. Nevertheless, considerable concern had been expressed that the "child's welfare" was such a vague concept that it allowed judges to decide cases purely on the basis of their own, perhaps idiosyncratic, views on family life. There were cases where mothers were favoured over fathers because the judge thought men should go out to work rather than stay at home to care for children; or where two-parent families were favoured over single-parent families. There were even cases where the judges gave their decision without explaining very clearly the reasons that had led them to choose one parent over the other.

In order to encourage judges to think more systematically, the 1989 Act sets out a "check-list" of matters to be taken into account when making decisions.[14] The courts must

have regard, in particular, to

(a) the ascertainable wishes and feelings of the child concerned (considered in the light of his age and understanding);

(b) his physical, emotional and educational needs;

(c) the likely effect on him of any change in his circumstances;

(d) his age, sex, background and any characteristics of his which the court considers relevant;

(e) any harm which he has suffered or is at risk of suffering;

31

(f)   how capable each of his parents, and any other person in rela-
        tion to whom the court considers the question to be relevant,
        is of meeting his needs;

(g)   the range of powers available to the court under this Act in
        the proceedings in question.

[s. 1(3)]

This check-list does not prevent any other matters being considered. Nor does it give any indication of how the items are to be
weighted. The order in which an item appears on the list has no particular significance. The fact that the "wishes and feelings of the
child" come first, then, does not mean that they carry any special
weight. Judges could discount them if they think that some other
consideration (whether or not it appears in the list) is more important provided that they make it clear that they are doing this. Nevertheless, it would be wrong if the judge totally ignored the child's
wishes, especially in the case of an older child.

How is the judge to find out what the child's wishes are? Judges
are divided over the desirability of meeting a child privately. If judges
do this, they must be careful not to make the child promises which
they cannot deliver (remembering that their judgment is always open
to appeal). Judges must also tell the adult parties anything the child
has told them which affects their decision. Although this could seriously inhibit children from indicating their views, the courts give
precedence to the fundamental principle of justice that the parties
should be able to comment on any item of evidence which might affect their case.[15] It is also accepted that talking to children about
such matters requires special skills, which judges do not necessarily
possess. The child's views, then, are most likely to be discovered by
the court welfare officer, since it is normal to request a report from
the court welfare service when parents are in dispute over the children. The officer should be careful not to put the child in the position
of having to choose between the two parents. This not only could be
damaging for the child, but also risks creating severe feelings of
rejection in the parent who is not chosen. But the welfare officer
must be sensitive to any strong indications of the child's preference,
and the reasons for this.

When divorcing parents have reached an agreement between
themselves about the ways in which their responsibilities are going
to be divided, it has been shown that courts are unlikely to investi-

gate the matter much further.[16] The courts can ask a welfare officer or a local authority social worker to report on any matters relating to a child's welfare in any case arising under the new Act [*s. 7(1)*]. But will they use this power if the adults have settled the matter between them? The new legislation seems to make this even less likely than under the law applicable before the Act. This is because, under the preceding law (*Matrimonial Causes Act 1973, s. 41*), a court could not make the divorce absolute (fully effective) unless the judge had certified that the arrangements proposed for the children were satisfactory or the best that could be devised in the circumstances. A judge might refuse to give a favourable certificate unless the welfare officer had investigated the situation. The 1989 Act repeals section 41. Now all that the court has to do is consider whether it should exercise any of its powers under the Act with respect to the children. Only if the court thinks that the circumstances require it, or are likely to require it, to exercise its powers, and if it is not in a position to exercise those powers without further information, *and there are exceptional circumstances which make this desirable in the child's interests*, can the court delay making the divorce decree absolute [*Sched 12, para. 31*].

The earlier power to allow the divorce to go through if the arrangements were the "best that could be devised" meant that courts did little to influence the arrangements made for the children. But it at least put on the parents the duty of presenting to the court a respectable set of arrangements. Although a person seeking a divorce will still have to declare the arrangements proposed for the children and usually attend an appointment with the judge, the judge will no longer have to evaluate the proposals and will now consider only whether to make an order or not. Indeed, when considering the arrangements, judges can ignore the check-list because they are obliged to consider the matters set out in the check-list (including the child's wishes) only if they are considering making a Section 8 Order *and the making of the order is opposed by any party to the proceedings* [*s. 1(4) (a)*].

If a child dislikes an agreement, there is no way in which his or her opposition can be formally communicated to the judge since the child is not party to the proceedings. It would, though, probably be unwise to ignore the child's views completely because this could be regarded as not giving proper attention to his or her welfare.

Of course, if parents have agreed about what is to happen to a child, a court's practical ability to *alter* these plans is limited. Nevertheless, the new restriction of the judge's power to take an overall view of the quality of the parents' decisions about what is to happen to the children is significant. This change is said to have been made in order to enhance parental responsibility.[17] It does seem to give the parents a freer hand than they, at least theoretically, had previously, but it is debatable whether this is encouraging responsibility or irresponsibility. The supervisory role of the divorce court will need to be re-assessed in the context of the anticipated proposals for the reform of the whole divorce procedure.

What will happen to people with orders made before the 1989 Act starts?

As soon as the 1989 Act comes into effect, *all* parents will acquire "parental responsibility" in the ways described in this chapter (so a divorced father whose ex-wife has "custody" of the children will have parental responsibility even if he has not been in touch with them for many years) but the *effects* of existing orders will be protected. Such a father will not be entitled to act inconsistently with any existing order. People who are not parents but who have "custody" or "care and control" under an existing order will also acquire parental responsibility, but can exercise it only consistently with any existing order [*Sched. 14*]. The basic principle is that, while the new concepts will apply where they can, people's *existing* rights will be protected. However, the interaction of the old and new laws could throw up technical legal problems and where they do come into contact, it would be prudent to obtain specialist advice.

Notes

1. This used to be referred to as "legal custody": Children Act 1975, s. 86: it is not mentioned in the 1989 Act, but who could doubt that it is still true?
2. Unlike some European countries, where parents may choose names only from a list approved by the state.
3. John Eekelaar, "The Emergence of Children's Rights" (1986) 6 *Oxford Journal of Legal Studies* 161; Jonathan Montgomery, "Children as Property?" (1988) 51 *Modern Law Review* 323.
4. Family Law Reform Act 1969, s. 8.
5. *Gillick v. West Norfolk and Wisbech Area Health Authority* [1986] AC 112.
6. See Andrew Bainham, *Children, Parents and the State*, London: Sweet &

Maxwell, 1988, pp. 52–3.

7. John Eekelaar, "The Eclipse of Parental Rights" (1986) 102 *Law Quarterly Review* 4.

8. For fuller discussions, see John Eekelaar, *Childright* 28 (June 1986) 9–10; Michael Freeman, *Childright* 51 (October 1988) 5.

9. *Dipper v. Dipper* [1981] Fam 31.

10. Law Commission, *Family Law: Review of Child Law: Guardianship and Custody*: Law Com. No. 172, London: HMSO, 1988, para. 3.14.

11. See John Eekelaar, Note (1988) 51 *Modern Law Review* 629, 630.

12. For an argument that the child's welfare should not be the sole consideration, see Pinhas Shifman, "The Welfare of the Child in Israeli Law – the Sole Consideration in the Laws of Minors?" (1989) 3 *International Journal of Law and the Family* 185.

13. Child Abduction Act 1985.

14. This is based on the proposals of the Law Commission. See Working Paper No. 96, para. 6.34.

15. *Elder v. Elder* [1986] 1 FLR 610.

16. G. Davis, A. MacLeod and M. Murch, "Undefended Divorces: Should Section 41 of the Matrimonial Causes Act be Repealed?" (1983) 46 *Modern Law Review* 121.

17. See Brenda Hoggett, "The Children Bill: the Aim" (1989) 19 *Family Law* 217, pp. 218–19.

Chapter three

A new framework for public law: local authorities and the courts

A society's commitment to protect children can throw up profound dilemmas. In theory at least, it is easy to pursue this goal when the society, or its appointed agents, and a child's parents are in agreement. But the whole position becomes more difficult when they disagree. A society could operate on a general assumption that children are best protected by their parents so that parents should be left alone to care for their children as they see fit. If, however, this were to be translated into the position that the protection of children and unrestricted parental control were the same things, the society would, in effect, have abandoned any claim to be treating children's interests as worth protecting in themselves. The only way to reconcile a commitment to child protection with respect for family autonomy is to accept parental care as being normally the most effective way of protecting and advancing a child's interests, but only so far as those interests, as defined by the wider society, are actually being advanced. In other words, a state committed to child protection can never accept family autonomy in child care as an end in itself. It is at most a means to an end.

In what circumstances and by what procedures should family autonomy be curtailed? As we showed in Chapter 1, in the past, the answer given in England and Wales depended largely on the force of circumstances. At the one end of the spectrum, a resolution might be passed through the social services committee of a local authority, without previous notification being given to the parents involved; at the other end, the elaborate paraphernalia of the High Court might be invoked under the "Rolls-Royce" procedure (as it was frequently called) of the wardship jurisdiction. Not only were the procedures different, but also the conditions that had to be proved to allow the displacement of the parents' rights differed according to the procedures chosen. The reform attempts to provide some coherence to this structure.

Under the new system, while a parent will be able to *share* parental responsibilities with a local authority under a voluntary arrangement, it will no longer be possible for the authority to acquire legal authority over a child without the parents' consent by a simple administrative act. This can now be done only by a court order. Moreover, it is intended that the *grounds* on which courts may intervene in this way should be clearly spelled out and that the grounds should be the same whatever the level of court in which the proceedings occur. These are the most significant changes introduced by the new legislation.[1]

Having decided that there should be no transfer of parental authority without the sanction of a court, the reformers attempted to rationalize the way in which these cases were handled. This chapter is primarily concerned with explaining how this has been done. However, it is also necessary to consider the *extent* to which courts do, and should, become involved in the decisions which must be taken in child protection work. To take the two extreme approaches – do we hand over the *entire* decision-making process to the courts or do we confine the judicial role to the periphery, allowing them to intervene only where things go seriously wrong with the administrative machinery? The reform displays some ambivalence over the nature of the appropriate relationship between the courts and social services departments. Since this relationship will be significant for the operation of the reformed law and its future development, we shall discuss it at the end of this chapter.

Care proceedings, family proceedings, courts and transfers between courts

The 1989 Act introduces a scheme whereby (1) compulsory acquisition of parental responsibility by a state agency (local authority) can be achieved only by a *Care Order*; (2) no *Care Order* can be made unless the local authority has applied for it; (3) the only method by which local authorities may *on their own initiative* seek a Care Order is by instituting *care proceedings*; (4) care proceedings can be brought in *any* court. The objective is to make *all* courts potentially available for care proceedings [*s. 92*]. However, Rules of Court may be made under the Act which could direct that certain types of cases could be *initiated* only in a particular court. Both the Lord Chancellor and the Solicitor-General have stated[2] that it is intended that care proceedings should always *start* at the level of magistrates' courts, but before the domestic, not the juvenile, courts and that those courts may *transfer* the case to a higher court if its complexity is such that this is considered desirable or to a similar court in a different location if it is thought that this will speed up the process.

There have been persistent calls for the Government to introduce a system of *family courts*, which would establish a single court in which all family matters would be dealt with. No firm Government decision has been taken on this. However, the 1989 Act could eventually lead in this direction. Under the Act, magistrates' domestic courts will be re-named "Family Proceedings Courts" and the Lord Chancellor is given power to regulate which types of proceedings brought under the 1989 Act and the Adoption Act 1976 should be dealt with at various "levels" of courts, including the County Court and the High Court, and to transfer cases within these levels. This means that the whole court system is potentially available for almost all family law business, and experience can be gained in the most effective ways of matching particular issues to particular courts [*s. 92 and Sched 11*]. But, although this imposes a conceptual unity on the system, the courts themselves and their administrators remain fragmented. The experiment may lead to the eventual unification of family law jurisdictions. It may also lead to greater complexity and confusion. An Inter-Departmental Working Party will be established to monitor its progress.[3]

Wardship proceedings

In Chapter 1 we gave a brief account of the nature of the wardship jurisdiction and how it came to be applied in cases of child protection. We referred to the growth of applications for wardship during the 1970s. This largely reflected dissatisfaction by local authorities with the scope and structure of care proceedings. The Working Party and the Law Commission were concerned that the continued existence of this jurisdiction could provide an avenue for either parents or local authorities to bypass the improved statutory scheme proposed in the *Review Report* and the *White Paper*. Both considered that wardship proceedings should effectively be removed as a means by which parental responsibility could be passed from parents to the state.

The 1989 Act achieves this by stating that a local authority can bring a case under the wardship jurisdiction only with special permission from the court. The judge can give this leave only if he or she is satisfied

(a)   that the result which the authority wishes to achieve could not be achieved through the making of any order of a kind (for which the authority is entitled to apply, assuming it is given leave to apply where this is necessary); and

(b)   that there is reasonable cause to believe that the child is likely to suffer "significant" harm if the court does not exercise its wardship powers.

[s. 100(3) & (4)].

The exact consequences of these provisions are a little uncertain and must await judicial interpretation. However, it seems that if the authority wishes to acquire parental responsibility over a child, or remove the child from home, these results could always be achieved through a Care Order made in care proceedings. Furthermore, if the authority wishes to challenge the exercise by a parent of any aspect of parental responsibility (such as providing, or refusing to provide, medical treatment), the authority can seek permission to apply for a Specific Issue Order [s. 10(2)(b)]; so, in either case, wardship would be unavailable. Furthermore, even if wardship proceedings are brought, the wardship court can no longer place the child in the care or supervision of the authority, nor can it require the child to be accommodated by it. Neither can the court give the authority greater powers than it already has. A child who is subject to a Care Order cannot be made a ward of court [s. 100(2)]. It is therefore difficult to envisage many occasions when the wardship jurisdiction would be useful for local authorities.

Nevertheless, such occasions may occasionally arise. For example, wardship might be useful if the authority wishes the court to control other people's behaviour towards a child (such as pestering by the press), to prevent a parent whose child is placed with foster-parents from harassing the foster-parents or, in an extreme case, even to obtain an order removing an adult from the home if this is in the child's best interests (see p. 93).[4] Another circumstance might be if the authority believes that it would be in a child's interests to undergo certain medical procedures. In *re F*.[5] the Court of Appeal suggested that there may be a *special category* of medical procedures, such as sterilization, abortion, or organ donation which, on account of their irreversibility, should be undertaken only with the permission of a court *even if the child's parents agreed to them*. The precise effect of the judgment is uncertain. Because of the *Gillick* judgments (see p. 24) it is unlikely that this applies if a sufficiently "mature" child consents to the procedure, unless the courts were to hold that a child can never be mature enough to agree to this category of action. The practical result seems to be that if an authority has parental responsibility over a child, these matters should always be brought before a court. If the child is on a Care Order, since it cannot be made a ward of court, the authority would need to apply for a Specific Issue Order (see below). If the child is not on a Care Order, the authority could seek leave to initiate wardship proceedings for the wardship court to take the decision.

In view of the limited occasions on which an authority might seek wardship, it seems unduly restrictive to allow its use only if the child is likely to suffer "significant" harm if it is not used. Why should it not be available in those few circumstances where it may be necessary to "promote the child's welfare"?[6]

Apart from the restrictions relating to local authorities, the wardship jurisdiction remains unaltered. Other organizations or individuals concerned with a specific child may still invoke the considerable powers which we described earlier (pp. 12–14). However, before the 1989 Act, the courts had held that, once a child had become subject to care proceedings, and especially if it had come into care under a Care Order, they would not allow the wardship jurisdiction to bypass the statutory procedures which had become applicable or allow the courts to take decisions for the child which had now been entrusted to the authority.[7] There is no reason to believe that this will change under the reformed law.

Applications for Specific Issue Orders and Prohibited Steps Orders

These orders were described on pp. 26–7. It is difficult to predict how significant they will become. For local authorities, they could replace wardship proceedings as an important alternative to care proceedings. If brought by an authority, the application will require prior permission, and it is likely that this will be obtainable only from courts above the magistrates' level. Neither order confers parental responsibility on a local authority, and the important decisions become the court's responsibility. For the same reason, the making of the orders is not dependent on proof of conditions necessary for making a Care Order. The court's decision is directed at the child's welfare as the "paramount consideration", taking into account the check-list set out in *section 1(3)* (se pp. 31–2). Nevertheless, the orders can place significant restrictions on the way a parent exercises parental responsibility. We will consider this further on p. 77.

If an authority has acquired parental responsibility, the Act specifically prohibits anyone using this procedure to question the way the authority exercises that responsibility [*s. 8(1)*].

Other family proceedings

When Care or Supervision Orders may be made

Although the reformed law confines local authorities' opportunities *to make an initial application for* Care or Supervision Orders to care proceedings, it may happen that concern arises about a child's welfare *during the course of* various types of family proceedings, such as divorce, adoption, maintenance or even wardship proceedings, or other cases where parents may be in dispute over the exercise of their "parental responsibility".

If this happens, and the judge thinks that a Care or Supervision Order might be an appropriate measure, he or she may direct the local authority to investigate the case and consider whether to apply for such an order. If the authority decides not to make an application, it must give the court its reasons and state what it is doing instead [*s. 37(3)*]. Of course, the court can make the Care or Supervision Order only if it finds that the conditions set out in *section 31(2)* (see Chapter 7) are present. If the authority decides not to make any application, the court itself cannot make a Care or Supervision Order, even if the judge would like to do so.

Family Assistance Orders

We have said that, in care proceedings, courts may make Care *or* Supervision Orders. The distinction between these will be discussed in Chapter 10. Under the previous law, a "supervision" order could also be made in divorce cases simply if the judge thought that there were exceptional circumstances which made an order desirable. In practice, judges made Supervision Orders for two rather different purposes. One was to make available to the parents the help of a welfare officer during the immediate aftermath of their divorce so as to ensure that the new living arrangements of the children would work out. The other was to keep an eye on a situation where there was some concern about the welfare of the children.

The new legislation separates these objectives. If judges are concerned about the children's welfare, they will be able to order an investigation by the local authority as described above and could make a Care or Supervision Order if the appropriate conditions (described in Chapter 7) are present. But if they simply think that the parents should be given some help in adjusting to the new situation, they can make a Family Assistance Order requiring a probation officer (divorce court welfare officer) or a local authority

> to advise, assist and (where appropriate) befriend any person named in the order.
>
> [s. 16(1)].

The order can name parents, anyone with whom the child is living or who has a Contact Order respecting the child, or the child personally. Since the point is to provide them with additional *help*, their consent is necessary before they can be named in the order, but if they are named, the order may require them to keep in touch with the assisting officer. To restrain excessive use of this power, the former restriction that it should be used only in exceptional circumstances is retained. Unless it is made for a shorter period, a Family Assistance Order will automatically lapse after six months.

Local authorities and abandoned children

If there is no one with "parental responsibility" for a child (for example, if the child is abandoned or orphaned, or perhaps if the parents become mentally incapable of exercising their responsibility), the local authority comes under a duty to provide the child with accommodation if it is needed [*s. 20(1)*] (see Chapter 5). But this does not give the authority parental responsibility for the child. Under the previous law, an authority might acquire "parental rights" in such circumstances by passing a resolution to that effect. It was the original intention of the reformers that an authority in this situation should be able to apply for a "guardianship order" [*White Paper*, para. 25]. But the 1989 Act has not carried this out. Although an authority has certain duties towards such a child (see p. 71), it would appear that there is no one with "legal responsibility" for the child, and that this cannot be achieved (other than through the child's adoption) unless an *individual* applies to a court for legal guardianship of the child (*s. 5*) or for a Residence Order (see Chapter 2). It is possible that a foster-parent could take one of these steps. The refusal to give a local authority the opportunity to acquire legal rights with respect to a child in these circumstances, unless it is at risk of significant harm (see Chapter 7), seems to be a further example of the hostility towards the acquisition of parental authority by state agencies which underlies much of the 1989 Act. Individual people must take responsibility for these children, or no one at all. Since the local authority does not have parental responsibility, it is unclear how far it can make long-term or significant decisions for the child beyond the mere provision of board and lodging.

Judicial review

For a number of years before the 1989 Act had been passed, the courts had shown a growing willingness to allow people whose interests were affected by local authority decisions to take proceedings in the High Court if they felt they had been unfairly treated by the authority. This procedure, known as "judicial review", has long been used as a way of keeping a check over the way government and other officials exercised their powers. We will discuss its details later (pp. 146–7). Here we will merely observe that its purpose is not to remove from officials their responsibility for making decisions but simply to ensure that they act fairly and follow the law when making them. The new law leaves this important supervisory role of the courts untouched.

The relationship between courts and local authorities

It is not easy to define the appropriate relationship between the courts and welfare agencies. There are, however, three main ways in which it could be structured. The first puts the court into the position of *decision-taker*. Under this model, the agencies are regarded primarily as collectors of information. This is then placed before a court which will decide whether the facts justify some intervention in the family and, if so, what form this should take. The second model sees the court as *referee*. Here the court is not necessarily thought to possess specialist expertise in the matters in issue. The responsibility for decision-making lies firmly with those agencies. But the court may be asked to decide whether the steps taken by the department in reaching its decisions were proper and provided a sound basis for action.

The third model defines the court as a *broker*. Under this model the court is actively involved in the negotiation between welfare agencies and parents, in an attempt to achieve an outcome which will at least be acceptable to all parties. It may, however, possess power to impose a solution should this be necessary. Such a court may well exercise some of the functions described in the previous two models, but adds to them an important new dimension in its stress on conciliation.

How, then, does the new legislation deal with the relationship between the welfare agencies and the courts? The first thing to note is that it confirms the leading role of local authority social services, who alone may bring care proceedings, although the NSPCC or some other body authorized by the Secretary of State may sometimes do so also [*s. 31(9)*]. The *Review Report* (para. 20), following the Select Committee, made a distinction between "major" issues "such as the transfer of parental rights and duties where there is or may be a dispute between parents and local authorities", which, it thought, should be "determined" by courts, and "case-management", which should be the responsibility of the local authority.

The problem is that it may be difficult to know where to draw the line between these two categories. The Working Party thought that decisions which might "impinge directly" on the "rights and duties" of parents and children fell within the first group, but recognized that decisions about contact between parents and children in care fell within both. In fact, many case-management decisions, such as whether to opt for long-term fostering, or whether to initiate a phased return home, could have consequences for the ultimate relationship between the parents and the children. In our view, the important decision to take is whether the issue is one on which it is appropriate for the court to *make a decision* or whether it is one which the court should only "referee".

Whether the circumstances set out in the law (discussed in Chapter 7) entitling a state agency to acquire parental responsibility exist must be a matter for *decision* by a court. It is for the courts to interpret the meaning of the legislative provisions, to decide whether the facts alleged (such as the "harms" claimed to have been suffered by the child) are established and to apply the law to the facts within the context of the community values in which they operate. Since it is probable that magistrates' courts in general reflect community values relevant to child protection more closely than do the higher courts, they will normally be the appropriate location for these decisions.

Once a court has decided that responsibility for a child should rest primarily with a welfare agency, the discharge of that responsibility lies primarily with that agency. It does not follow that this should be free from external supervision. However, we would argue that, at this stage, the court, if it is to act at all, should follow more closely the "referee" model.

This is for two reasons. First, the types of decisions made after the initial intervention seldom involve the ascertainment of facts and the application of law to such facts, but are usually open-ended evaluations of what actions are most likely to promote the welfare of children. Neither magistrates nor judges have the training or experience in child care to make detailed decisions of this kind and it seems improbable to suppose that they can be given these skills. Even if judges and magistrates were retrained, it would be contrary to principles of good organizational management to remove the power to make day-to-day decisions from those who have to provide the resources necessary to give effect to them. Child care must have sufficient flexibility to respond to the needs of the child, to innovate and to abandon unsuccessful measures before they can cause harm. Furthermore, the cost to social services' time of having to engage in courtwork on a large scale could seriously undermine resources available for casework as well as subverting morale and motivation by apparently removing the responsibility of decision-making from social services personnel to the courts.

But our main reason is constitutional. Decisions about child care management reflect judgments about the ability of social and health services to control, predict or monitor behaviour and the extent to which public resources should be committed to these purposes. Since these are ultimately political decisions, it is right that they should be open to debate and ultimate control within the political sphere. Social workers are answerable to their superiors within the department and the department as a whole is, in principle, answerable to the locally elected council, and potentially liable to investigation through public inquiry. The 1989 Act establishes a procedure for complaints about the way local authorities are looking after children [*s. 26(3)*] (see p. 147). Ultimately, of course, the Government, which is answerable through Parliament to the electorate, is responsible for the thrust of child care policy, which it implements through legislation, circulars, administrative arrangements and, most of all, the provision (or non-provision) of resources.

It is important to contrast this with the position of the courts. Their independence is premised on the theory that they should not be accountable, except perhaps in the most extreme cases of incompetence, to a political body, nor their decisions subjected to public inquiry or a complaints procedure. Lower courts must, of course, follow the law and ascertain the facts as correctly as possible, and the appeal system is designed to correct errors. But decisions about child care are not susceptible to the same kind of analysis as legal judgments. Indeed, when the higher courts do make decisions about children's interests, such as deciding which parent should look after a child after divorce, the internal checks within the appeal system are very limited.[8]

Of course it is true that many of these considerations apply to the initial decision whether or not to intervene legally into a family. It is a feature of child protection law that issues occur across a continuum and do not easily break down into neat categories. But it has long been accepted that, where the law allows the executive to intervene in important ways in people's lives, it is the unique role of the courts to decide whether the conditions permitting such intervention have been satisfied, irrespective of the implications for policy or administrative convenience. This is a cornerstone of the idea of the Rule of Law.

But once that threshold has been crossed, the role of the courts becomes more problematic. In asserting that, if the court is to become involved at this stage, it should be as a referee rather than a decision-maker, we leave open the question of the extent to which it is desirable to refer such decisions to the courts *at all*. At the one extreme, it could be alleged, as is suggested in the *Review Report*, that *every* decision which might have substantial consequences for the child should be taken to a court, at any rate, if requested by some interested party.[9] Up to now, however, only certain kinds of decisions are selected for this treatment. If it is understood that in these cases the court is to adopt the role of decision-taker, the objections to referring such issues to them we have outlined apply fully. If, however, the court acts only as referee, the objections lose some (but not all) of their force. The undesirability of diverting social work resources into courtwork would remain.

Limitation of the involvement of the courts may be achieved either by restricting the *types* of decisions referable to them, or by narrowing the *grounds* upon which local authority actions can be reviewed by the courts. During the debates in the House of Lords on the Children Bill, the Lord Chancellor made it clear that he appreciated many of the points we have been making concerning the relationship between the role of the courts and of social services.[10] It is perhaps for this reason that the 1989 Act adopts both these techniques for restricting court involvement in child protection decisions. Only certain specified issues (notably, those concerning contact between children in care and their parents) may be referred to a court which can substitute its own decision for that of the local authority. Other actions taken by the authority affecting children in its care and their parents are susceptible to "judicial review", but this is restricted to ensuring that the authority has acted in a fair and rational way.

Our evaluation of the reformed structure therefore is that in principle the enhanced, and improved, judicial role at the point of legal entry within the family accords with the proper relationship between the courts, state and citizens which we have described, although, as will appear, we have some reservations as to its application to emergency situations. In principle, we believe that the role of courts *after* initial intervention should be circumscribed. Although the Act does place some limitations on such involvement, we believe that these may not be adequate and that this may turn out to be an unsatisfactory area which will require further attention.

Notes

1. See speech of the Lord Chancellor, *House of Lords Debates*, vol. 502, cols. 489 and 493 (6 December 1988).
2. See *House of Lords Debates*, vol. 502, col. 494 (6 December 1988) (The

Lord Chancellor) and House of Commons, Standing Committee B, 8 June 1989, col. 462 (The Solicitor-General).

3. See *House of Commons Debates*, vol. 158, col. 553 (23 October 1989) (The Solicitor-General).

4. See *re T.* [1987] FLR 181.

5. (1989) 138 *New Law Journal* 183; on appeal, the House of Lords approved the principle that it was desirable that the permission of the court should be sought prior to a sterilization on an adult who could not give consent due to mental incapacity; the House confined its observations to sterilization operations: *F. v. West Berkshire Health Authority* [1989] 2 All ER 545.

6. Nigel Lowe, "Caring for Children" (1989) 139 *New Law Journal* 87.

7. *A. v. Liverpool City Council* [1982] AC 363; *re W.* [1985] AC 791.

8. See *G. v. G.* [1985] 2 All ER 225 (House of Lords).

9. Lowe op. cit.

10. See *House of Lords Debates*, vol. 503, col. 1521 (7 February 1989).

Chapter four

The organizational context of child protection practice

In order to understand how child protection work is likely to be affected by the 1989 Act, it is important to appreciate the distinctive characteristics of the principal agencies involved. This chapter will discuss their work and consider the problems in achieving satisfactory co-operation between them.

Social services departments

Social services departments occupy the central position in the working of child care law and their role will be examined in detail in later chapters. The key to understanding their approach, however, is to recognize that they are organized in an essentially bureaucratic fashion. The notion of 'bureaucracy' has been rather disparaged in recent years. Much of this criticism misses the point. As a form of organization, bureaucracy emerged alongside modern states as the "great chain of command" from rulers to citizens. With the spread of representative democracy, it became an instrument for the administration of those rules which citizens themselves had drafted to regulate their own society. One may criticize the practical imperfections, but something like a bureaucracy is an inevitable consequence of the sort of collectively provided services that we enjoy in a welfare state, making a link between those who are paying for services and those who are consuming them.

What this means, in practice, is that social services departments are organized in a fashion which is designed to reflect their accountability to elected representatives. This may be undercut by the inertia of electors or councillors, or by the unionization or professional aspirations of social workers but it is none the less a basic operational principle.

Local government social work, then, places considerable weight on the defensibility of its decision-making. This comes through in a number of ways. The two most important here are record-keeping and supervision. All social work decisions are elaborately documented and held on file for possible review. Thus it can be a matter of some significance whether a child is already known to the department by means of a file, and whether that file relates only to the child or deals with the whole family and various adult problems. Moreover, if a referral is made in writing, it will have to be filed and, since a record of contact has been created, some action will have to be documented, even if only a letter of acknowledgement. Telephone contacts have a much more ephemeral existence and cannot force the organization to respond with anything like the same effect. This attention to record-keeping is related to the close supervision of fieldworkers, with the object of ensuring that their practice conforms to departmental policy, that it does not incur financial or other obligations and that it does not exceed the department's legal powers or duties. Responsibility is constantly being transmitted upwards. Basic-grade social workers have relatively little discretion compared with, for example, general practitioners (GPs) or even health visitors.

These factors have an important influence on social services' response to reports of children in possible need of care or protection. There are two common complaints about this: of precipitate action and of undue delay. These may seem merely to suggest that social workers are in a "no-win" situation, but both can be accounted for by features of departmental organization. GPs, for instance, sometimes complain that, having notified social services of a child about whom they are concerned but whose case they wish to handle themselves, the department has immediately initiated its own investigation. The department, however, is under a statutory duty to make such inquiries. (The effect of the 1989 Act on this duty will be discussed on pp. 82–3). This places the onus on the referrer to give as full an account of the cause for concern and his or her intended action as is possible. That account will, of course, have to be in writing. Even then, its adequacy is a matter for the judgement of the social services rather than the referrer.

The second complaint can also be related to the demands of public accountability. Other than in a few well-defined emergency situations, referrals to social services must go through a vetting and allocation process. To the referrer, of course, all referrals are urgent, but the department has to ration its time and resources by looking at referrals in competition with one another. This is a problem which GPs, in particular, have, in the past, seldom encountered, in the absence of effective cash limits on their practice costs. Once again, the force of referral is greatly enhanced if it is in writing and can, to some degree, speak for itself rather than through the mediation of a duty officer.

Social workers themselves are a very heterogeneous group. Many of the senior staff qualified before the advent of generic training and have specialized backgrounds in child care, mental welfare, almoning and the like. More recent entrants have come via both graduate and non-graduate routes. The former are again divided between those who have done accredited undergraduate degrees and those who have obtained postgraduate qualifications. So while the basic licence, the Certificate of Qualification in Social Work (CQSW), is the same, its substantive content varies considerably. Few departments have been able to fill all their social worker posts with qualified staff. The service went through much more comprehensive reorganization than any other agency during the 1960s and early 1970s, and the subsequent period of relative stability has seen increasing financial constraint. Inevitably there has been a great deal of confusion, debate and turmoil over the basic nature of the occupation's mandate.

The health services

The general approach of health service personnel can be examined in relation to the legal duties on the Secretary of State for Health to promote a national health service designed to ensure the 'improvement ... in the physical and mental health of the people' in England and Wales and to provide such facilities 'for the care of expectant and nursing mothers and young children as he considers appropriate as part of the health service'.[1] In the 1984 case of Heidi Koseda, who was shut in a room in her home and starved to death, an officer of the relevant health authority was reported as saying that they did not have an *in loco parentis* relationship to her.[2] While it is true that the health authorities did not stand in a parental relationship to Heidi, nevertheless health service personnel are employed in the furtherance of the Secretary of State's duty to improve the health of the people. Even if they do not have the power to carry out this duty in the face of opposition, for example, by entering property against the wishes of the occupier, or removing children, they can comply with it by referring the matter to others who do have or can acquire those powers.

Community health services

Community health staff are employees of District Health Authorities (DHAs). The changes which have resulted from the Report of the Griffiths Inquiry into NHS management in 1983[3] make it very difficult to give a general picture of the organization of community health services. While most authorities seem to have grouped medical and nursing staff into a community unit for management purposes, there is considerable variation in the influence of professional concerns on the precise structure adopted. However, it seems to be common for a Specialist in Community Medicine to retain an important role in providing clinical and policy leadership on child health. He is also likely to be responsible for a staff of clinical medical officers, who will provide health surveillance through the authority's child health clinics and school health services. In recent years, however, these services have tended to decline in favour of greater GP involvement in the routine monitoring of children's growth and development. Community nurses – health visitors, district nurses, school nurses and, occasionally, community midwives – still tend to have a separate line of management, to a Director of Community Nursing. Some areas, though, have tried to introduce territorially based management, merging medical and nursing lines, while others have considered basing their units on care groups, so that a unit manager might be responsible for all services to children, whether in hospital or the community.

Staff in other agencies need to bear in mind the low level of integration in child health services. All of the occupations involved have strong and jealously guarded traditions of autonomous practice. This is as true of community health services, with their apparently bureaucratic structures, as it is of GPs under their independent contracts. This means, for instance, that people should not assume that if they give information to GPs it will also go to their attached nurses, or vice versa. The same applies to communication within community health services and the flow of messages between field-workers and managers. The amount of management influence on community nursing seems to vary considerably. Some areas have tried to reduce this in the name of giving more clinical autonomy to field staff. Others, responding to the findings of some of the child death inquiries about the weakness of supervision in community nursing, have cut down the amount of discretion they allow and tried to impose much more uniform policies.

Health visitors

Health visitors are registered nurses with recognized obstetric training who have completed a one-year certificate course (HV Cert). This course combines academic instruction, in psychology, sociology, social policy, social epidemiology and health visiting principles, with supervised practical experience. There is also a small number of graduates from nursing degrees which include components accepted as equivalent. Most health visitors are women. Their caseloads tend to be high. The 1972 DHSS recommendation of one health visitor to 3,000 population is rarely approached, and ratios go as high as one to 10,000 and more in some metropolitan districts. This translates into caseloads of anywhere between 250 and 1,000 individuals, most of whom will be children under five. All births are routinely notified and the family visited at home. Traditionally, these visits would continue at intervals determined by the health visitor until the child reaches school age. It is difficult to generalize about these home visits but, typically, they last about twenty minutes. In the course of this time, the health visitor attempts to make some assessment of the home environment and each child's physical, emotional, cognitive and social development, and to respond to any problems raised by the child's caretaker (almost invariably the mother). In any one year, health visitors see around 70 per cent of all children under five, including almost every newborn baby, in their own home.

Recently, however, this practice has been changing in some areas. A number of authorities have been trying to link visiting schedules to risk-assessment scoring, despite the limited evidence for the validity of any such tool. It does, though, produce more statistical information which is thought to be helpful in planning the distribution of resources. Some authorities have also been influenced by the libertarian ideas discussed in Chapter 1 to reduce the extent of home visiting generally and unannounced visiting in particular. Their health visitors are used much more on clinic-based work with less direct community surveillance. Priorities are determined by available public data on needs rather than the search for individual cases.

In areas where such developments have occurred, health visitors have reduced their uniquely favourable position for identifying the needs of young children. Where it remains, their combination of knowledge about both physical and social factors in growth and development bridges the gap between doctors and social workers, who tend to specialize in one or the other. Health visitors as an occupation have a vast experience of looking at normal children in ordinary homes, which helps them to recognize signs or symptoms that might be overlooked by people with less representative experience.

Despite their lack of coercive powers, health visitors' traditional work pattern of unannounced home visiting allows them to conceal any special interest they may have in a child. If there is concern about a child's nutrition, for instance, a health visitor can 'accidentally' call at mealtimes. This can be very useful in cases where anxiety about a child's welfare has not crystallized into a clear basis of evidence which might justify the firm identification of a need for care or protection. Wherever there is concern about a child under five, it is advisable to consult the relevant health visitor at an early stage. Indeed, if the child who is causing concern is over five but has siblings below that age, it is still likely to be worth involving the family's health visitor for what she can offer on the history and current state of the household. Conversely, if such surveillance is not going on, it is important that other agencies do not assume that it is and become lulled into a false sense of security.

Community midwives and district nurses

Other community nurses may occasionally become involved in child protection. The most important of these are community midwives. Health authorities vary somewhat in the way in which the care of mothers and babies is divided between midwives and health visitors. In general, however, midwives carry out home visiting of new mothers from their confinement, or hospital discharge, until the tenth day after birth. Antenatal visiting forms part of their duties in some areas and they are also empowered to follow cases for up to twenty-eight days after birth. This clearly gives them an opportunity to monitor a child's home circumstances and the quality of care he or she is receiving. On the other hand, this contact is probably too short to be of great value except in alerting other agencies to possible problems. Its most obvious uses are likely to be in identifying the need for various sorts of voluntary intervention such as assistance with housing or care for other children during confinement or illness in pregnancy. Where a pregnant woman is under sixteen and unmarried, the question may arise as to whether she should come into care in her own interests, which might also allow for more effective protection of her baby.

District nurses also have a minor role in child protection. Some of their work is with sick children where concern might develop about their parents' ability to provide continuing care. They are also occasionally used to monitor children in a household where they are ostensibly nursing an old person. A clinical reason for frequent visiting may be more acceptable to the family than a high level of health visitor surveillance.

General practitioners

Primary care services are provided by GPs who are independent contractors rather than employees of the NHS. This means that GPs enter into an agreement to provide primary medical care for people registered with their practices. In return, they are paid a basic annual fee for each registered patient, weighted by age, and additional fees for undertaking certain specific tasks like family planning or antenatal care. Historically, their focus has been on the treatment of ill-health, either by their own prescriptions or by onward referral to specialists based in hospital. There have, however, been moves towards a more preventive orientation. Many GPs have taken over the provision of routine child health services from community medical staff. Most community nurses are now attached to general practices, although they remain accountable to the health authority. Community nurses work with rather than for general practitioners.

GPs tend to see children in clinics or surgeries, rather than at home. The numbers involved are quite substantial: every year about three-quarters of all children under fifteen will visit a GP for some illness, averaging four to five consultations each; and about 80 per cent of all children under one year are seen at clinic sessions, although that falls off quite sharply to less than half of two- to five-year-olds. However, it is only with the recent development of vocational training for GPs that they have had any specific preparation in the knowledge and skills of child health work and there are still large numbers of self-taught older practitioners around. Even so, it is hard for any GP to match the degree of social understanding and the experience of normal children possessed by health visitors working along traditional lines. This is a very important point for people in other agencies. There is an inevitable tendency to accept medical opinions without questioning their basis. At the same time, community nurse reports are often discounted, despite their possibly greater validity.

Child health and school health services

Theoretically, these services provide a parallel system for the general screening of children's health and development until school leaving age. Where disorders of growth or behaviour are identified, children should be referred for more specialized intervention, referrals which may bring them into the care and protection system. Responsibility for under-fives, however, has increasingly passed to GPs and child health clinics now tend to play a residual role, except in those areas where the primary care services have been unable or unwilling to take on the work. The school health service is widely recognized to be in a rather unsatisfactory state. It relies heavily on part-time staff, both doctors and nurses, whose knowledge and commitment are less than complete and whose efforts are often poorly organized and ill co-ordinated. Some areas have been trying to improve matters and there are, of course, many individuals with a considerable depth of interest and concern. Nevertheless, much will depend upon these unpredictable local variations as to the contribution which either service can make on any particular occasion.

Accident and emergency departments

Accident and emergency departments see large numbers of children – between a quarter and a third of all patients are under fifteen. However, the work is unpopular with doctors and the departments are particularly dependent on overseas-trained staff and on those who are required to obtain accident and emergency experience as part of their specialist training in surgery. Because of differences in cultural background, the former may have great difficulty in assessing British-born children. The latter are looking towards careers in general or orthopaedic surgery rather than paediatrics. In consequence, accident departments tend to have a narrowly clinical focus, responding to the presenting injuries rather than making the broad appraisal of a child's general condition which is the first step in considering the possibility of a need for care or protection. Paediatric accident departments staffed by doctors with appropriate knowledge of, and interest in, child health are found only in a few urban areas.

An important, but often unrecognized, contribution could be made by nurses or other locally recruited staff, like receptionists or ambulance crews, in making rather wider assessments of a child's condition in relation to his or her social environment. Unfortunately, there is often no institutional channel through which this can be communicated, especially if the medical staff are insensitive to its possible relevance.

Hospitals

Most hospital specialties can impinge on children's welfare in their treatment plans for adult patients. The admission of an adult to hospital may mean a child's coming, temporarily or permanently, into local authority care. These implications can easily be overlooked in concern for the adult involved. Sometimes, the child's interest is at stake more directly. This is perhaps most obviously the case in obstetrics, where decisions about the clinical management of childbirth may have implications for the mother's perception of her baby and their ability to form a satisfactory relationship with each other.

Wherever children are permitted to visit, ward staff have an opportunity to observe parent–child interaction. There are a few occasions on which this could be significant. For instance, where a woman has been admitted with injuries suspected, but not acknowledged, as resulting from a beating at the hands of a husband or cohabitee, observation of her children might be important in deciding whether there is some threat to their health or welfare. On children's wards, of course, the patients have been admitted because they are in need of health care. If there are welfare issues, these are already likely to have been identified, although ward nurses may be able to collect further data. One case which has arisen was where a child, who had come into hospital with unexplained gastric and neurological symptoms, failed to respond to treatment. When observed, the child's mother was seen to administer tablets to her and it was revealed that the symptoms resulted from deliberate poisoning.

The medical specialty most involved with children is, of course, paediatrics. Its central focus is the health of children, their illnesses and disorders of growth or development. Along with the parallel specialty of child psychiatry, its contribution is likely to be crucial in any case which involves the physical or mental state of a child. Where such a case has arisen, the relevant doctors should be brought in at an early stage to make a comprehensive and authoritative examination of the child if there is any possibility, however slight, of legal action. If possible, this examination should be carried out by a consultant, or at least a registrar, rather than a house officer. Legal intervention may prove unnecessary, but this should ensure that the decision for or against proceeding is taken with adequate clinical evidence available.

People from other agencies often find hospital medical staff easier to deal with than GPs. In part this reflects the more hierarchical organization. Once some policy is agreed with the consultant, then he is likely to ensure that it is followed by his junior staff. There may be frustrations. Initial contacts may be with relatively inexperienced doctors who have difficulty in establishing exactly what is expected of them. It is important, then, that the referrer gives as much background information as possible and is able to point to the implications of the clinical findings and the standards they may have to meet as evidence. Access can also be a problem if the child's GP is obstructive. Sometimes it is possible to make referrals through community medical staff. A few paediatricians will accept 'under the counter' referrals from health visitors and social workers. One possibility is to use a referral to child guidance, which can lead to a child psychiatrist and thence to a paediatrician. In an emergency, of course, an injured or sick child may be taken directly to an accident department.

Police surgeons

Mention should also be made of the work of police surgeons. Most of these doctors are GPs who have received some specialized training in forensic work and are available to be called out when the police require medical assistance in their work. There has been considerable controversy about their role in child protection cases.

While it now seems to be generally accepted that victims of physical abuse or neglect should be examined by paediatricians, who will then provide any evidence necessary either for care proceedings or for a prosecution, the responsibility for sexual abuse cases is still contested as the debates over the Cleveland Report have underlined. This partly reflects the greater emphasis placed on criminal prosecutions in such circumstances and the division of opinion about whether such events are better treated primarily as a form of abuse or as a form of rape.

Problems of liaison and communication

The management of children in need of care or protection can be an extremely complex organizational problem. A variety of workers with widely differing social and intellectual backgrounds and embedded in quite different sorts of agency structures must, somehow or other, communicate information and co-ordinate action.

The problems of liaison between them have frequently been identified by public inquiries as causes of errors in case management.[4] In the *White Paper* (para. 43) the Government stated that it would "make legal provision for co-operation between statutory and voluntary agencies in the investigation of harm and protection of children at risk". The 1989 Act therefore *requires* local authorities, local education authorities, local housing authorities, health authorities and other persons (to be designated by the Secretary of State) to assist an authority which is investigating suspected abuse [*s. 47(9) (11)*] as long as the assistance sought is "not unreasonable" [*s. 47(10)*]. It also requires those agencies, so far as compatible with their statutory duties, to assist any local authority which calls upon them for support in the exercise of the authority's general powers and duties towards children (described in Chapter 5) [*s. 27*]. It should be noted, however, that the legislation requires the relevant agencies *to respond to initiatives taken by the local authority*. There is no *reciprocal* duty laid upon local authorities to respond to approaches made by other bodies, unless the approach triggers a duty already laid upon the authority (such as the duty to investigate suspected harm under under s. 47). It is arguable that full co-operation is unlikely to be achieved unless some such duty were to be created (such as, for example, a duty to consider *all* reports received from certain sources, to take such action as appropriate and communicate this and the reasons for it to the reporting agency). We discuss this further on p. 83.

Apart from any statutory provisions, most areas have responded to the problem by attempting to develop some sort of inter-agency liaison system. The details vary greatly but certain features tend to be common. These include the existence of an Area Child Protection Committee (ACPC), the operation of a Child Protection Register and the use of local case conferences.

Area Child Protection Committees

Area Child Protection Committees (formerly called Area Review Committees) bring the agencies together at the top. They were created and developed under the influence of a series of DHSS circulars from 1974 onwards. The system was reviewed by the department during 1987 and new advice, *Working Together*, was issued in 1988 about arrangements for inter-agency co-operation in child abuse cases.[5] ACPC members are generally chief officers or their deputies from health, social services, education, probation and the police. An ACPC will probably meet as a body only two or three times a year, but various subcommittees will come together more frequently. The ACPC attempts to co-ordinate policy formation in the constituent agencies. It will issue an inter-agency procedure handbook which attempts to set out each agency's responsibilities and approach for the benefit of its own staff and those liaising with them. *Working Together* emphasizes that ACPCs should keep these handbooks under constant review. (Appendix 6 sets out a recommended standard form for such handbooks.) The document also advises ACPCs to make an annual review of the child protection work done in their area and to plan for the coming year. ACPCs may organize interdisciplinary training sessions and are also likely to oversee the local child protection register, whichever agency actually keeps it.

If the ACPC is to be a workable body, however, certain major difficulties must be overcome. Since it lacks any statutory basis, it is largely dependent on the goodwill of constituent agencies for its resources, although the recent linkage to the Joint Planning arrangements between the health service and local authorities has eased this problem. More importantly, the lack of any statutory base complicates the enforcement of decisions. How can member agencies be sure that each will follow the agreed guidelines? Because each agency has distinct objectives and duties, each must reserve the right to disregard collective decisions in the light of its own responsibilities. ACPCs vary considerably in the degree to which this is seen as a purely theoretical possibility, so that departures in any agency from agreed policies will normally lead to internal disciplinary actions. The closer a committee approaches this position, the more effective its work appears to be. Nevertheless, as the *Cleveland Report* showed, there continue to be difficulties in establishing this degree of collective responsibility in some areas.

The most unified ACPCs have developed systems for the active monitoring of fieldwork practices. These tend to be based on panels of managers drawn from the core agencies – community medicine and nursing, social services, police, NSPCC. The panels may operate largely on a paper basis, receiving and reviewing reports from case conferences, but some areas have used them as a kind of permanent case conference with fieldworkers attending to present and discuss particular cases.

Child Protection Registers

One of the most important functions of the ACPC is its oversight of the local Child Protection Register (CPR). *Working Together* introduced this new title for what used to be called At-Risk Registers as part of its attempt to clarify their role and function. In the past the addition of a child's name to the register was frequently thought to do no more than indicate concern. A child's name could remain on the register simply as a "flag" rather than with the implication that it was subject to special attention. A CPR, however, is now defined as a list of children who are currently the subjects of specific interagency plans for their protection. The data to be held on the register should include (apart from details about the child, its immediate carers and the nature of the harm involved) the name and telephone number of the key worker assigned to the case, the child's doctor and health visitor, the programme set out for dealing with the case and the schedule for reviewing the programme. In particular, it is the intention of the Department of Health that the progress of action regarding children on the register *should be formally reviewed every six months* (*Working Together*, para. 5.32).

A child's name will normally be entered on the register only after a case conference which has been attended by all the relevant agencies.[6] If the conference decides to recommend legal action, the child's name should go on the register, even if only to record the arrangements about where the child will live and the basis on which contact by parents or others may take place. Many entries, however, are likely to be made when proceedings are not immediately planned. *Working Together* recommends that registration should take place if a child has been harmed. It could also be appropriate to place the child's name on the CPR if there is serious concern about the treatment of another child in the same household. A child should be removed from the CPR only with the agreement of another case conference.

The judgment of the High Court in *R. v. Norfolk County Council, ex parte M* [7] raises serious issues for social services departments when they contemplate making an entry on the CPR. If the department wishes to enter the name of an individual on the register as the actual or alleged abuser, it will need to adopt a "fair" procedure. Unfortunately, the court did not specify precisely what procedure had to be followed other than to say that what was fair depended on the circumstances and was a matter on which reasonable opinions might differ. The department has to make a genuine attempt to reconcile its duty of child protection with a duty of fairness to the alleged abuser. While this is a matter on which social services departments should seek guidance from their legal departments, we would suggest that the action taken should be influenced by the *consequences* for the (suspected) abuser of registration. These were serious in the *Norfolk County Council* case because the department communicated their suspicions to his employer. If it is desired to do *no more than to* record a suspicion, it may be unnecessary to go further than recording clearly that the individual is only a suspect, what the grounds for suspicion are and that the person has not been given a chance to refute the allegation. The courts will be slow to intervene in such a way as to inhibit placing the child's name on the CPR.[8] If, on the other hand, the registration reflects a belief in a person's guilt, or if actions which may prejudice the individual are likely to follow from the registration, it may be necessary to involve the legal department so that the matter can be raised with the individual, either directly or through solicitors.

Working Together recommends that the register should be established and maintained by the local social services department, or the NSPCC on its behalf, and managed by an experienced social worker with special skills in child abuse work. The Department of Health and the Welsh Office hold lists of CPR custodians for England and for Wales. In principle, anybody working for a recognized agency should be able to telephone a central number to ask whether a child is known to be on the register. This facility is particularly important for emergency or out-of-hours services where the history implied by registration may be a crucial element in the interpretation of suspicious but inconclusive evidence from other sources. The inquirer should be provided with the name of the child's key-worker but it is probably unwise to give out other information over the telephone. Inquirers should make their own professional judgement on the facts available to them. If the child about whom an inquiry is made is not on the register, a record should be kept of its name and of the advice given. It is important to check if there is a child on the register living at the same address.

Specialist Assessment Teams

The *Cleveland Report* recommended that local authorities should establish Specialist Assessment Teams, consisting of a senior social worker, an approved medical practitioner and a police officer to which cases of sexual abuse could be referred. Referrals could be made as soon as any practitioner or agency suspected abuse had occurred and the team would control any further assessment or investigation. This approach might also have some merits in cases of physical abuse although the relationship between such teams and case conferences would need to be carefully worked out. *Working Together* (para. 6.11) recommends that ACPCs explore the suggestion.

Other devices designed to promote better inter-agency communication

The *Review Report* had little to say about organizational issues in child care and concentrated heavily on legal questions. Legal changes, though, achieve their effects only through the organizations which implement them. Deficiencies in organizational systems have been repeatedly revealed by both academic research and public inquiries. Yet, apart from the suggestion of establishing Specialist Assessment Teams for cases of sexual abuse, little has been done other than to urge agencies to improve arrangements for co-operation and communication. This is clearly something which has had only limited success over the years. Two changes were considered and rejected.

Power to initiate proceedings

One option was to increase the powers of agencies other than social services departments to deal directly with cases. For example, under the old law, the NSPCC and the police had the power to initiate care proceedings independently of the local authority. Even the local education authority could do this, although in practice this was normally limited to school non-attendance cases. The Working Party thought there was no reason why the police should retain this power, or for education authorities to have it, except in school non-attendance cases, and this is now the position under the 1989 Act.[9] However, *s. 31(9)* allows the NSPCC to bring proceedings on its own initiative and permits the Secretary of State to license other bodies to do this [*s. 30(1)*], although they will now be obliged to consult the social services department in advance [*s. 31(6)*].

The *Review Report* paid little regard to the role played by health services in the detection of cases of child abuse and neglect. Yet there might be a case for giving local health authorities power to initiate care proceedings, or at least to initiate a procedure which would compel the authority to explain to a court why it was *not* taking action. The report's emphasis on the dominant position of social services seems to have prevented it considering such a possibility. Only social services, it was argued, could judge whether voluntary intervention was feasible and determine what facilities it was "willing to make available" to meet the requirements of any court order (*Review Report*, paras 12.5–16).

But this argument is not conclusive. Once an authority has reasonable cause to suspect that a child in its area is suffering, or is likely to suffer, significant harm (and this must almost always be the case if it is so informed by the health services) the authority must decide whether to take any action to safeguard or promote the child's welfare [*s. 47(1)*]. As we point out in Chapter 6 (p. 83), this formulation represents a diminution of the authority's duty as it stood under the previous law, which obliged them to bring proceedings where the defined grounds appeared to exist unless they were satisfied that this would not be in the public interest or that of the child. Now the authority may just decide to do nothing. In such an event it could be useful if designated bodies (such as health services) were expressly given the power to force the authority's hand. There is a rarely used legal procedure for compelling public authorities to perform their statutory duties called an application for *mandamus*, but this is so unusual as to be irrelevant to child welfare law. There might be a case, then, for the creation of a simple procedure within the framework of child welfare law whereby the issue of whether the child was suffering significant harm could be raised in a court by parties other than the local authority and the social services department required to explain what they proposed to do about it. Such a power, even if seldom used, could have the organizational consequence of encouraging health services to systematize their collection of information, social services to pay closer attention to referrals and both to improve their channels for mutual communication (see *White Paper*, para. 43).

Reporting abuse and neglect

The other device which might have been used in the new legislation to press for closer inter-agency co-operation would have been the introduction of a legal obligation on any person, or specified groups of people, to report formally to social services any information leading them to suspect that a child was being abused or neglected. The Working Party discussed this idea but rejected it. It thought that a "reporting law" might raise "barriers between clients and their professional advisers", and "set back the advances made over the years in encouraging inter-disciplinary communication and co-operation" (*Review Report*, para. 12.4). A law of this kind was unnecessary because most of the professionals who might be affected by it were employed in the public sector and subject to its employment discipline in observing agreed voluntary reporting procedures. Moreover, they were imbued by a strong emphasis on "welfare" from their training (*Review Report*, para. 12.3). But the problem lies less in attitudes towards welfare, than in conflicting traditions of professional independence. The professionals may all want to do good, but have different conceptions of what that is and how it might be achieved.

Nevertheless, we think that the Working Party was right to reject the introduction of mandatory reporting laws in the context in which it was working. The fact that health service and voluntary organization personnel do not have coercive powers plays an important part in the establishment of relationships which allow them to investigate cases at a low level of suspicion without antagonizing clients. A mandatory reporting law would inevitably link these personnel with the more threatening powers of local authorities. It seems right, then, that the decision to retain or pass on information should rest upon their professional judgement.

It must be noted, however, that one of the reasons for the prevalence of reporting laws in the USA is the complications introduced into child protection work by the existence of large private and charitable sectors in health and welfare. Doctors treating children privately at the expense or under the insurance of their parents may need to be reminded that their duty is to their patient rather than to the person who is paying the bills. Welfare agencies operating within a particular ethnic or religious group may be pressed to collude with abuse out of group loyalty. If there is a substantial change in the pattern of health and social service provision, the case against a reporting law may become much weaker. The proposals for NHS reform, for example, envisage that GPs will be subjected to much greater consumer pressures which will tend to run against the assumptions about the force of their duty to the "public good" on which voluntary notification is based.

Privileged access to information

In *D. v. NSPCC*[10] the House of Lords decided that the NSPCC was entitled to withhold the identity of people who informed it about cases of suspected child abuse or neglect even from a court. There was a public interest in the efficient operation of the child protection machinery, and if the NSPCC did not have this privilege, its sources of information might dry up. While it is probable that this protection would be extended to other agencies, if the matter came before the courts again, this cannot be absolutely certain. It would have been useful if the 1989 Act had taken the opportunity to extend this principle to all reports made to any agency involved in child protection work.

A related issue could also have been dealt with. If anyone passes on information to an appropriate authority (such as the police, or agency personnel), suggesting that a child might be experiencing abuse, that person is protected against possible libel proceedings by the parents if he or she acted in good faith. In spite of this protection, however, the possibility that bad faith (mischief-making) might be alleged, putting the reporter at risk of trouble, expense and legal proceedings to establish their integrity, might deter people from reporting reasonable suspicions. Teachers are said to be particularly worried about this. The law *could* help by conferring *absolute privilege* on reports of child abuse made to specified authorities by certain classes of people, like teachers or health workers. This would mean that no legal action could be taken against such reports in any circumstances.

Notes

1. National Health Service Act 1977, s. 1 and s. 3.
2. See *The Times*, 26 September 1985.
3. *NHS Management Inquiry* DA (83) 38, London: DHSS 1983.
4. See Chapter 1, Note 5 and *Report of the Inquiry into the Death of Doreen Mason*, Area Review Committee for Lambeth, Southwark and Lewisham, 1989.
5. DHSS, *Working Together: A Guide to Arrangements for Inter-Agency Co-operation for the Protection of Children from Abuse*, London: HMSO, 1988.
6. The exception would be if a registered child moves into the area from elsewhere.
7. [1989] 2 All ER 359.
8. *R v. Harrow London Borough Council ex parte D*, [1989] 2 FLR 51.
9. The police do retain an independent power to remove a child to safety in emergencies (see p. 93).
10. [1978] AC 171.

owers and duties of local
horities: family support and
preventive action

The most significant ways in which a modern society helps its children are to be found in its general services for promoting the health, education and welfare of the population. Viewed somewhat narrowly as a process of keeping people from falling into need, this area of policy and practice is sometimes described as primary prevention. Secondary prevention occurs when people meet specific problems which threaten to undermine their ability to provide adequately for themselves. Its objective is to offer short-term assistance in order to "prevent" those at risk from falling into longer-term dependence on state provision. In the case of children, this usually means some form of local authority service.

The general powers and duties of local authorities respecting children

The Working Party was dissatisfied with the legal framework in which English and Welsh local authorities carried out their preventive policies. On the one hand, under section 1 of the Child Care Act 1980,[1] there was a general duty on every local authority

> to make available such advice, guidance and assistance as may promote the welfare of children by diminishing the need to receive children into or keep them in care under this Act or to bring children before a juvenile court.

Thus the duty to "diminish the need to receive children into care" was owed to *all* children. In carrying out this duty, the authority had the power, if it thought fit, to give assistance "in kind or, in exceptional circumstances, in cash".

On the other hand, local authorities had overlapping powers, and sometimes duties, under a range of other statutes to provide services or facilities which could benefit specific groups of children. For example, local authorities were under a duty to provide special facilities for people who were blind, deaf or dumb or otherwise substantially and permanently handicapped,[2] and were permitted to provide services for the prevention of illness or the care of persons suffering from illness.[3] Local authorities differed widely in the way they classified expenses between those arising from their powers under section 1 of the 1980 Act and those associated with other forms of community or residential aid.

The Working Party felt that all these functions should be brought within a single legislative framework as they affected children. But it did not think that they should all be merged into section 1 of the 1980 Act. Its wording seemed to be too negative because it directed authorities only to reduce the prospects of children coming into care (which might be interpreted as simply "keeping families off their books") rather than stressing the positive value of family support.

The Government accepted this view [*White Paper*, para. 22a]. Local authorities should no longer be under an obligation to diminish the need to receive children into care, although they should remain under a duty to diminish the need to take children into care *compulsorily*. Local authorities were to be given a "broad 'umbrella'" of *powers* to provide services to promote the care and upbringing of children, and to help to prevent breakdown in family relationships (*White Paper*, para. 18). In analysing how these intentions have been carried through in the 1989 Act a distinction can be drawn between *all* children and those children defined by the Act as *children in need*.

Duties and powers with respect to all children

The duties which local authorities owe to *all* children in its area are

1 to "take reasonable steps designed to" reduce the need to bring care, criminal or other family proceedings relating to them, to encourage them not to commit offences and to avoid the need to place them in secure accommodation

[*Sched 2, Pt 1, para. 7*]

2 to "take reasonable steps" through the provision of services mentioned in Part III of the Act, "to prevent children within their

area suffering ill-treatment or neglect"

[*Sched 2, Pt 1, para. 4(1)*]

3 to "provide such family centres as they consider appropriate" where families may attend for various activities, including advice

[*Sched 2, Pt 1, para. 9*]

4 to "take reasonable steps" to identify the extent to which there are children in need in their area; to publish information about the services provided and to take such steps as are reasonably practicable to ensure that those who might benefit from these services receive the information.

[*Sched 2, Pt 1, para. 1*]

Although apparently covering *all* children within the local authority area, the Act states that these duties are imposed on local authorities for the "principal" purpose of enabling them to discharge their obligations to children who are "in need" [*s. 17(2)*].

In addition to these duties, local authorities are given certain *powers* which may be exercised in favour of *all* children in their area, even if not "in need". Authorities *may* provide (1) day care for such children under five who are not at school [*s. 18(2)*]; (2) facilities (including advice and training) for people caring for children in day care [*s. 18(3)*]; (3) "care and supervised activities" for school-age children outside school hours and during holidays [*s. 18(6)*]; and, (4) accommodation for any child within their area (even though a person with parental responsibility can also provide it) if they consider that this would safeguard and promote the child's welfare and for those aged between sixteen and twenty-one in a community home if they consider that this would safeguard and promote the child's welfare [*s. 20(4) and (5)*].

The provision of accommodation under *section 20* is an important power and will be discussed in more detail on pp. 74–9.

Duties and powers with respect to children in need

Once a child is identified as being "in need", additional duties are imposed on the authority. The Act states that

... a child shall be taken to be in need if

(a)   he is unlikely to achieve or maintain, or to have the opportunity of achieving or maintaining, a reasonable standard of health or development without the provision for him of services by a local authority under this Part;

(b)   his health or development is likely to be significantly impaired, or further impaired, without the provision for him of such services; or

(c)   he is disabled.

[*s. 17(10)*]

"Development" means physical, intellectual, emotional, social or behavioural development, and "health" means physical or mental health [*s. 17(11)*]. It will be noticed that this includes children who may not yet be suffering any harm, but who are likely to do so unless something is done.

Authorities are put under a *general duty*

(a)   to safeguard and promote the welfare of children within their area who are in need; and

(b)   so far as is consistent with that duty, to promote the upbringing of such children by their families, by providing a range and level of services appropriate to those children's needs.

[*s. 17(1)*]

In order to carry out this policy, authorities are put under a variety of specific duties. The only unqualified duties towards children "in need" which are placed on a local authority are

1   to open and maintain a register of disabled children within its area [*Sched 2, Pt 1, para. 2*];

2   to inform a different local authority if it believes that a child within its own area is likely to suffer harm but lives or proposes to live in the area of that other authority [*Sched 2, Pt 1, para. 4(2)*];

3   to provide services for the disabled [*Sched 2, Pt 1, para. 6*];

4   to provide accommodation for any child in need who appears to require accommodation because he has no one parentally responsible for him, or has been lost or abandoned, or whose carer cannot suitably look after him, or who is sixteen (but under eighteen) and the authority thinks the child's welfare is likely to be seriously prejudiced without such provision [*s. 20(1) and (3)*].

71

As already mentioned, the duty to provide accommodation will be discussed further on pp. 74–9.

Other duties towards children "in need" are qualified. These are the duties

5 to "take reasonable steps", where a child in need is living apart from his family, to enable the child to return to his family or keep in contact with his family, if, in the authority's opinion, this is necessary to safeguard or promote his welfare [*Sched 2, Pt 1, para. 10*];

6 to "make such provision as they consider appropriate" for various services (such as advice, occupational and recreational activities, home help and assistance towards holidays) to be made available for children in need who are living with their families. [*Sched 2, Pt 1, para. 8*].

7 to provide day care "as is appropriate" for children in need within their area who are under five and not yet attending schools [*s. 18(1)*].

In addition, a local authority is given the *power* to assess the needs of a child in need for the purposes of the 1989 Act at the same time as any assessment of needs is made under various other Acts, such as the Chronically Sick and Disabled Persons Act 1970 [*Sched 2, Pt 1, para. 3*].

Enforcement of powers and duties

There is, as will be noticed, a careful gradation between duties and powers. What is the significance of drafting the Act in this way? One object is clearly to signal a set of priorities to local authorities. Efforts are to be directed primarily at (1) averting *compulsory* intervention (including diminishing delinquency); then, (2) taking reasonable steps to identify particularly vulnerable children and to prevent neglect and abuse and, (3) "targeting" resources on such children (particularly the disabled and those without accommodation). There is, however, a good deal of subjectivity in the definition of the children to be targeted.

Legally, however, the distinctions are less significant. An individual who has a particular interest in the matter may bring proceedings, either personally, or sometimes through the Attorney-General, asking a court to declare that a local authority has made improper use of a statutory power or duty. This applies to *failures* to act as well as to inappropriate actions. In some circumstances, then, it is possible for an authority to be ordered by a court to take some particular action, and it is possible that it would be legally wrong for an authority to adopt a policy which prevents it from discharging a duty.[4] A court might decide that an authority was not acting unreasonably even if it made no attempt whatsoever to exercise a power, whereas, in the case of a duty, the authority would have to show that it had, at least, made reasonable efforts (given its resources) to comply.[5] However, if a duty is expressed in very wide terms, such as the general duty in section 17, or is hedged around with qualifications, such as that "reasonable steps" must be taken, all a court can do is to consider whether the authority's actions are a reasonable way of implementing the purposes for which it was imposed.

The same is true if someone is physically injured by the negligent exercise of a power or a duty, or by the negligent failure to exercise a duty. The injured person (say, a child who had suffered abuse and who claimed that this was the result of the failure of the authority to perform a duty) may seek to sue the authority concerned for compensation. But it is difficult to prove negligence and such remedies are useful only in exceptional cases. They do not provide a satisfactory method for the routine monitoring of authorities' use of their powers and duties.

The practical result is to place this responsibility on the political process. This seems to be appropriate. The means by which families are supported are extremely varied and it would be difficult for a court to determine what the "best" mix might be. However, there are potential points of conflict between local and central politicians. The most obvious is the retention in the 1989 Act of local authorities' power to give assistance "in kind or, in exceptional circumstances, in cash" [*s. 17(6)*]. This may overlap with the role of central government agencies. Under the Social Security Act 1986 discretionary payments for people experiencing "exceptional needs" may be made from the Social Fund administered by local offices of the Department of Social Security. These payments are means-tested and may take the form of loans rather than grants. The Government intends such payments to be confined to severe emergencies, such as where someone loses cash, or experiences theft, fire or flood. It is not difficult to imagine that some authorities may choose to make more generous cash payments under the 1989 Act than would be available

73

under the Social Security Act 1986. Others, however, may take advantage of their new power to provide loans rather than grants to adopt a much more restrictive approach [*s. 17(7)*], but loans cannot be made to people receiving income support or family credit under the Social Security Act 1986 [*s. 15(9)*].

The provision of day-care for children under five has proved controversial. The Act carefully distinguishes between such provision for *all* children and for children in need. Local authorities *may* provide for the former, but *must* provide for the latter "as they consider appropriate" [*s. 18(1) & (2)*]. Neither is a particularly strong directive, and in an attempt to meet criticism, the Government inserted a section requiring authorities to review their day-care provision, together with the availability of private child-minders, at least once every three years [*s. 19*].

It should be noted that local authorities have power to contract-out the provision of services [*s. 17(5) (b)*] and may recover a "reasonable charge" for any service provided, other than advice, counselling or guidance, from a child's parents or, if the child is over sixteen, from the child [*s. 29(1) & (4)*].

The provision of accommodation

One of the main objectives of the 1989 Act was to restore the sense that a voluntary relationship between local authorities and families in difficulty could be a positive measure. Voluntary care, in particular, had assumed a more "threatening" aspect as a result of the pressures on local authorities during the 1970s to adopt a more cautious approach to the return of children to their parents. The Children Act 1975 had included a provision that allowed authorities to require twenty-eight days' notice from the parent before handing back a child who had been in care for six months or more. The House of Lords had also ruled that, even before the six months' period had elapsed, a child did not automatically cease to be in the authority's care the moment a parent asked for his or her return. Nor did the authority have a duty to give back the child if it thought this was against the child's interests.[6] Unless the parent removed the child by self-help, the authority could continue to hold the child and pass a resolution under the Child Care Act 1980, s. 3, assuming parental rights.

The Working Party tried to weaken this increasingly sharp distinction between being in and out of care. If finer gradations could be devised and used imaginatively, care might play a useful supplementary role in helping families in difficulty. The Working Party came up with proposals for two new legal statuses, which they called *respite* and *shared* care. Respite care was modelled on the experience of giving short-term relief to families with a handicapped child by taking the child into residential or foster care for a limited period. If a child were in care for less than a month, parents could simply delegate their day-to-day responsibility for the child to the authority, but could reclaim the child at any time without having to give notice. Shared care would involve an agreed transfer of legal responsibility for the child from parents to the local authority. Parents would need to give twenty-eight days' notice to end this arrangement so that the authority could plan the child's return. The authority would, however, be obliged to exercise this responsibility only in consultation with the parents.

The Government did not accept the Working Party's proposals completely. It thought that the distinction between respite care and shared care was not "readily sustainable in practice" and concluded that "it would not be helpful to make this distinction in law" (*White Paper*, para. 26). Instead, it proposed that "matters such as initial placement, schooling and access and subsequent changes to these arrangements should be settled by mutual agreement" (*White Paper*, para. 23). It also decided to abolish the existing requirement for twenty-eight days' notice before a parent could reclaim a child after he or she had been in care for more than six months. Local authorities would, however, still be free to make this part of their agreement with parents when a child was received into care. The authorities would also lose the power compulsorily to acquire parental rights by administrative means. This could now take place only through care proceedings, as we discuss in the next chapter.

Section 20 implements these policies. It abandons the conceptual language of being "in care" and replaces it with the practical language of "providing accommodation". Fieldworkers and other practitioners must grasp that, henceforth, *the expression "care" is to be confined to the context of compulsory intervention*. Voluntary arrangements between an authority and parents are viewed as a kind of "back-up" to parental care which the parents can *choose* and *repudiate* as they wish. Children looked after by an authority under such arrangements should probably be referred to as "accommodated children". *Section 20* states:

> Every local authority shall provide accommodation for any child in need within their area who appears to them to require accommodation as a result of
>
> (a) there being no person who has parental responsibility for him;
> (b) his being lost or having been abandoned; or
> (c) the person who has been caring for him being prevented (whether or not permanently, and for whatever reason) from providing him with suitable accommodation or care.

[*s. 20 (1)*]

This provision imposes a duty to provide accommodation not only for abandoned or orphaned children but also for children whose carers are unable to care for them. But even if a child's parent is able to look after him or her, and the child is not "in need", the authority *may* accommodate the child if it thinks this would safeguard or promote the child's welfare [*s. 20(4)*]. A parent is allowed to "arrange for some or all of his parental responsibilities" to be met by "one or more persons acting on his behalf" [*s. 2(9)*], and this would cover such an arrangement with the authority. But in *either* case (that is, whether the parent was able or unable to care for the child), the whole arrangement hinges on the parents' agreement, since the Act also states that

> Any person who has parental responsibility for a child may at any time remove the child from accommodation provided by or on behalf of the local authority under this section.

[*s. 20(8)*]

So someone with parental responsibility may remove an "accommodated child" even if this is in breach of an arrangement with the authority. No notice need be given, even if this was stipulated in the agreement. The question may well arise in the courts after the Act is brought into force, but we think that a court will decide that it would be against the policy of the Act to use contractual remedies to enforce an agreement under which a parent restricted his or her rights, protected by the Act, to look after the child. It is, then, unlikely that a court would, for example, grant an injunction to prevent the parent from moving the child.

What, then, is an authority to do if it believes that it would be against the child's interests to return to the parent? The authority could consider the following options:

1 It might consider applying for an Emergency Protection Order, followed, perhaps, by a Care Order (discussed in Chapter 6). But these are extreme measures and require evidence that the child is likely to suffer significant harm if returned, and that the harm would be occasioned by the parents' failings. It may be that the social workers believe that the harm to the child will result more from being upset by a precipitate removal than the quality of the parents' care, and wish to do no more than to reintroduce the child into his or her family by a phased, planned process. So these measures might fail.

2 It might consider initiating wardship proceedings. These, as we have described (pp. 38–40), would require permission from the court. But this may be refused because the result desired by the authority (a phased return of the child) could be achieved under a Care Order and it may not be possible to demonstrate that the child is likely to suffer "significant" harm if the jurisdiction were not invoked (see p. 40).

3 Finally, the authority might apply to a court for permission to seek a Specific Issue or Prohibited Steps Order (see pp. 26–7). Remember that no Residence Order may be made in favour of a local authority [*s. 9(2)*]. This seems much more likely to succeed. The authority need show only that it is in the child's best interests (by the "paramountcy" test: see pp. 30–1) that an order be made, and the order can require the parent to exercise his or her responsibility as directed by the court. This could presumably include a direction that the parent should allow the child to remain in local authority accommodation.

However, even if the authority were to acquire an order in those terms, it may yet be faced with the difficulty that *section 20(7)* states clearly that an authority "may not" provide accommodation for any child if a person with parental responsibility, who is willing and able to provide accommodation, or arrange for its provision, objects. If the parent is not "able and willing" to provide, or arrange, accommodation for the child, the authority will retain its power to accommodate the child. But although this will legitimize the authority's continued retention of the child, it will not override the parent's right to remove the child under *s. 20(8)*, so the parent will always be able to come and take the child away.

Section 20(7) makes no reference to the *quality* of the accommodation offered by the parent or the circumstances prevailing there. So, provided accommodation of some kind is available, and the parent wants the child back, the authority loses its legal power to keep the child. Even if an order were to prohibit a parent from removing the child, it is not clear that this section would be overridden and that the local authority could lawfully use its resources to accommodate the child. This problem will probably have to be solved by the courts. It is unfortunate that the emphasis placed on safeguarding parental responsibility from encroachment by welfare agencies should have left such uncertainty in a significant matter.

Although we think it probable that an agreement between a parent and an authority will not be legally enforceable as if it were a contract, this does not mean that the fact that an agreement has been broken by a parent will have no practical significance. The breach could form an important part of the authority's case if it feels compelled to apply for an Emergency Protection or other Order or, ultimately, a Care Order, as evidence of the unreliability of the parent (see Chapter 8).

If an authority is looking after a child with the agreement of a residential guardian (see p. 30), or of someone who has care of a child under an order made in wardship proceedings, then, so long as that person wishes the child to remain with the authority, no parent or other person with parental responsibility can remove the child [*s. 20(9)*]. The residential guardian or person with care can, of course, remove the child at any time.

Another situation where the parent cannot compel the return of the child is where the child is sixteen and wishes to stay in local authority accommodation [*s. 20(11)*]. In fact, it is possible that the House of Lords' decision in *Gillick v. West Norfolk and Wisbech Area Health Authority*[7] means that the wishes of an even younger child could prevail over those of a parent in these circumstances. If, as the judgment implies, "parental rights" disappear when a child achieves sufficient understanding and maturity to make his or her own decision on some matter, a parent may well lose the legal power to direct where a child is to live before the child reaches sixteen. More detailed negotiation of the terms under which an authority "provides accommodation" for children seems likely to constitute an increasingly important part of the social services' approach in child welfare work. The loss by the authority of two important statutory powers (the ability to impose a twenty-eight days' notice on reclamation of a child and the power to pass a resolution assuming parental rights) marks a significant shift in the bargaining strength of parents and the authority. For example, under the twenty-eight days' notice system, an authority could put pressure on parents to agree to a phased return of the child, at least over that period. Now an authority may have to threaten to use drastic coercive measures (such as an Emergency Protection Order) or contemplate court proceedings to achieve what they think is best for the child. In trying to reduce the distinction between voluntary care ("providing accommodation") and *not* being in care, the reformed legislation has sharpened the line between voluntary and compulsory action.

General duties of local authorities to children looked after by them

A local authority can find itself looking after children in a variety of circumstances with somewhat different legal implications. In Chapter 10 we shall examine the position of children who come into this position as a result of a Care Order. Here we shall refer only to the core duties owed to all children for whom an authority provides accommodation for more than twenty-four hours, whether under a voluntary arrangement or under a court order. These are the duties

(a) to safeguard and promote his welfare; and
(b) to make such use of services available for children cared for by their own parents as appears to the authority reasonable in his case.

[*s. 22(3)*]

The child is to be treated as similarly as possible to children who are living with their own parents. Moreover, the authority must, in regard to any matter to be decided respecting the child, so far as is reasonably practicable, ascertain the wishes and feelings of (1) the child; (2) his or her parents; and (3) any person who is not a parent of the child but who has parental responsibility for him or her and (4) any other person whose wishes and feelings the authority considers to be relevant [*s. 22(4)*]. Having ascertained those wishes, the authority must give them "due consideration" and must also give "due consideration" to the child's "religious persuasion, racial origin and cultural and linguistic background" [*s. 22(5)*].

It has been suggested[8] that the duty to "safeguard and promote" the child's welfare is less favourable to children than the duty the previous law placed upon authorities to "give first consideration to the need to safeguard and promote the welfare of the child throughout his childhood" [*Child Care Act 1980, s. 18*]. We feel it unlikely that the new wording will have practical significance. The new statutory duty is directed at the child's welfare, not that of any interested adult. However, the abolition of the concept of "care" except in the context of compulsory intervention, and the re-casting of the role of the welfare authorities as no more than a "back-up" provision, with ultimate authority retained clearly in the hands of those with parental responsibility, will make it more difficult for the authority to implement measures it may think necessary to safeguard the child's welfare.

A new scheme of registration

Parts 6–11 of the 1989 Act contain important new provisions relating mainly to the registration and regulation of community homes provided by local authorities, voluntary homes run by voluntary organizations, children's homes, private fostering and day care and child-minding. These fall outside the scope of a book intended primarily as a practical guide for fieldworkers. However, the new provisions up-date and rationalize many old statutes. Stricter controls are placed over private fostering, such as the number of children allowed to be fostered, notification by parents of intention to arrange the fostering of their children and the disqualification of certain people from carrying out private fostering. As far as child-minding and day care are concerned, the main change is to concentrate regulatory efforts on provisions for children *under the age of eight*. People who look after such children for money for periods exceeding two hours in any day need to be registered with the local authority. Nannies are exempt. Local authorities will now be *required* to impose such requirements on the registered person, for example, as regards the keeping of records, the number of children to be minded and the maintenance of premises and equipment as they consider appropriate. The 1989 Act also for the first time imposes a duty on persons in charge of independent schools to safeguard and promote the welfare of children who reside at the school and on local authorities to ensure the duty is complied with [*s. 87(1)*].

Notes

1. This derived from the 1963 Act discussed on p. 17.
2. The Chronically Sick and Disabled Persons Act 1970, s. 2.
3. National Health Service Act 1977, Schedule 8.
4. There is an extensive body of law on the question; see for example S.A. de Smith, *Constitutional and Administrative Law*, Harmondsworth: Penguin, 1985, ch. 28; see *Attorney-General, ex rel. Tilley v. Wandsworth London Borough Council* [1981] 1 All ER 1162.
5. See *R. v. Bristol Corporation, ex parte Hendy* [1974] 1 WLR 498.
6. *Lewisham London Borough v. Lewisham Juvenile Court Justices* [1980] AC 273.
7. [1986] AC 112.
8. Christina M. Lyon, "Legal Developments following the Cleveland Report in England – a Consideration of some Aspects of the Children Bill", (1989) *Journal of Social Welfare Law* 200.

Chapter six

The acquisition of compulsory powers: first steps

It would be wrong to suppose that the use of compulsory powers implies that positive family support has been abandoned. There may be occasions when the threat of the compulsory measures may succeed where persuasion has failed to achieve the removal of a threat to a child (for example, from a dangerous cohabitee). This is especially so now that (as we shall explain in Chapter 9) the range of compulsory powers has been broadened under the new laws. Nevertheless, as we have seen, the 1989 Act directs local authorities to act in ways which will diminish the need for compulsory intervention [*Sched 2, Pt 1, para. 7*]. But, of course, such occasions will arise. When should voluntary measures be replaced by compulsory ones?

The duty to investigate and consider

A full answer to this question will involve an analysis of the new grounds for bringing care proceedings, which we shall set out in Chapter 7. For the present, we shall just look at the general framework. As we have seen (p. 44), local authorities are the main initiators of care proceedings. Under the previous law, local authorities had a *duty* to bring proceedings if there appeared to be grounds for doing this, unless they thought that neither the child's *nor* the public's interest would be served by doing so [*Children and Young Persons Act 1969, s. 2(2)*]. The reformed law has, curiously, removed this duty.

Under *section 47*, when a local authority is informed that a child in its area is subject to an Emergency Protection Order (EPO), or is "in police protection" (these situations will be discussed on pp. 85–93), or when it has reasonable cause to suspect that a child in its area is suffering, or is likely to suffer significant harm or where the authority has obtained an EPO with respect to a child,

> the authority shall make, or cause to be made, such enquiries as they consider necessary to enable them to decide whether they should take any action to safeguard or promote the child's welfare.

$$[s.\ 47(1)\ \&\ (2)]$$

The new law obliges the authority to put itself in a position to decide only *whether* it should take action to safeguard or promote the child's welfare (for example, by seeking a court order). The Act does later go on to say that, if the authority decides it should take action, then it must take it [*s. 47(8)*], at least so far as it is within its power and is reasonably practical for it to do so, but that does not put it under an obligation to decide *that it should* take the action, even if it believes that the child has suffered, or is likely to suffer, significant harm. As the law is worded, it seems possible that a local authority, having made its enquiries, could decide *against* taking action because, for example, it did not have adequate resources or intervention might provoke political or ethnic pressure groups. The authority could even make no decision at all simply through inertia.

Although this issue was not specifically discussed in the *Review Report*, there was no indication of any intention to dilute the former duty to initiate care proceedings. The position now, however, seems to be that the presence of a duty to *reduce* the need to bring care proceedings coupled with the absence of a duty to take such proceedings even where a child is in danger might be taken to signal political coolness towards the use of compulsory measures. Whether this (if it is indeed the case) translates into practice remains to be seen. We would hope that authorities would see it as their duty to take whatever action they deem necessary (within the Act) to safeguard a child's welfare whenever their enquiries reveal that the child's welfare is in jeopardy.

The Act contains a number of provisions to help social workers carry out enquiries on behalf of their employer. For example, it is stated that any local authority, local education authority, local housing authority or health authority is under a duty to assist the enquiring authority, unless the request is unreasonable. If necessary, the Secretary of State can be asked to place any other person under a similar duty [*s. 47(9), (10) & (11)*]. Investigation is to be thorough.

The 1989 Act states that, in carrying out the enquiries, the child should be seen, usually by a social worker, unless the authority believes it already has sufficient information; and if it is refused access to the child, the authority should apply for an EPO, a Child Assessment Order (see pp. 90–2), a Care Order or a Supervision Order unless it thinks the child's welfare can be adequately protected without doing this [s. 47(4) & (6)].

Emergency protection

There are, inevitably, occasions when immediate compulsory intervention is necessary to protect a child until a full court hearing can be held. Under the old law, this was done by obtaining a "Place of Safety Order" which involved the applicant (usually the local authority) asking a magistrate for authorization to detain the child for a specified period (the maximum was twenty-eight days) in a safe place. Anxiety had been expressed during the 1970s over the increasing number of applications for Place of Safety Orders (which were very rarely turned down), although there was no hard evidence that inappropriate applications were common. Indeed, such applications were rare events for both social workers and juvenile court magistrates [*Review Report*, Annex C, para. 6]. Nevertheless, various informal safeguards had been built into local procedures. In some areas, applications were sifted by the magistrates' clerk. But the most common way of restraining the use of the procedure was by granting orders for a period much shorter than the maximum permitted.

In fact, the technical defects of the procedure were probably a more important reason for change than any evidence of abuse. Strictly speaking, an order could not be made unless a child was actually being harmed at that very moment. There was also some doubt about whether an order could be made if a child was already in a safe place like a hospital or residential home (the order authorized the child to be "*taken*") even if the child's removal from there would be dangerous. Moreover, it was not clear whether an order gave doctors any right to *investigate* (as distinct from treat) a child's condition. Yet many children held on Place of Safety Orders in Cleveland were subjected to investigation and questioning regarding suspicions of sexual abuse.[1] It was also unclear whether the parents of a child held on a Place of Safety Order could be denied access, something which became a major problem in the Cleveland cases.

In an attempt to deal with these difficulties, the 1989 Act abolishes Place of Safety Orders and replaces them with Emergency Protection Orders (EPOs) and Child Assessment Orders (CAOs).

Emergency Protection Orders

Conditions upon which EPOs may be granted

On receiving an application, a court may make an EPO with respect to a child if it

is satisfied that there is reasonable cause to believe that the child is likely to suffer significant harm if

(a) he is not removed to accommodation provided by or on behalf of the applicant; or
(b) he does not remain in the place in which he is then being accommodated.

[*s. 44(1)(a)*].

The Act speaks of a "court" making the order, but it is intended that regulations will enable applications to be made to a single magistrate outside court hours in emergencies.[2]

A court may also make an EPO if the local authority or an "authorized person" (the NSPCC) is investigating suspected abuse and find that their access to a child is being frustrated by unreasonable refusals to allow the child to be seen, provided that they have reasonable cause to believe that such access is urgently required [*s. 44(1) (b) and (c)*].

If an EPO is made, anyone in a position to do so must hand the child over to the applicant *if asked*. The applicant, who will normally be a local authority, is then authorized to accommodate the child and prevent his or her removal from wherever he or she happens to be, such as a hospital ward. It should be noted that, although medical personnel may *advise* against the discharge of a child from hospital, they have no legal authority to prevent it unless an EPO is in force. The applicant acquires parental responsibility over the child [*s. 44(4)*], but no one else loses their responsibility. Even if an EPO is in force, the applicant may still allow a child to stay at home and must, in any case, return the child as soon as this can safely be done.

Medical assessment

The EPO allows the applicant only to

> take such action in meeting [its parental] responsibility as is reasonably required to safeguard or promote the welfare of the child (having regard in particular to the duration of the order) and shall comply with the requirements of any regulations made by the Secretary of State for the purposes of this subsection.
>
> [*s. 44(5)*]

This seems to limit medical (or other) actions to those necessary for the child's immediate welfare. If the applicant can foresee that additional diagnostic work might be needed, this must be stated *when applying for the EPO*. The court can then give

> such directions (if any) as it considers appropriate with respect to ... the medical or psychiatric examination or other assessment of the child.
>
> [*s. 44(6) (b)*]

If the authority overlooks this point when applying for the EPO, or finds that these powers are necessary after the order has been made, it can go back to the court and ask for an appropriate extension [*s. 44(9)*]. But the child's parents will also be able to ask for the directions to be varied at any time. The court granting the EPO can also "impose conditions" when making the order and these might include a direction that there should be *no* medical or psychiatric examination or assessment, or none unless a court subsequently approved [*s. 44(8)*]. It is obviously desirable, therefore, that a local authority should be as thoroughly prepared as possible when it applies for an EPO if it expects that further diagnosis and assessment of the child will be necessary. Indeed it may be a good idea to ask for the power to examine the child for the purposes of assessment as a matter of routine in all cases. But additional court-based work is likely to occur as a result of these changes and all agencies must incorporate this into their resource planning and case management arrangements. Fieldworkers should note that, in accordance with the *Gillick* principle (p. 24), a child of sufficient understanding can refuse to submit to examination or assessment [*s. 44(7)*]. It could be argued that the child's interests might best be served by examination because there could be cases involving older children who have been intimidated by an abusing parent into refusing consent and that the harm to the child could be revealed only by forcing the child to submit to examination.[3] But most cases of physical or even sexual abuse where medical evidence will be crucial will involve children too young to fall within the "maturity" test of the *Gillick* judgment (see p. 24). In our view, the right of a mature child to bodily integrity should be accorded priority. Any other view could amount to authorizing (further) physical or sexual assault on the child.

Contact between children on EPOs and their parents

The *Review Report* had suggested that the entitlement of parents to access to a child held under emergency powers should be defined more clearly. If, for any reason, an authority thought it was undesirable for a parent to visit the child, social services should ask the magistrate for permission to refuse visits and, if necessary, to conceal the child's address. This matter became more urgent as a result of the events in Cleveland and is taken up in the 1989 Act. When a child is being held under an EPO, the applicant must still allow "reasonable contact" with the following people: the parents (this includes an unmarried father who does not have parental responsibility); anyone who has parental responsibility for the child; anyone with whom the child was living immediately before the EPO was made; anyone in whose favour a Contact Order is in force with respect to the child and anyone acting on behalf of those persons [*s. 44(13)*].

Since the whole point of the order may well have been to protect the child against just those people, authorities may often have good reason to fear the consequences of such contact. As with medical assessments, they must anticipate this when they make the application, since the magistrate or court may make

> such directions (if any) as it considers appropriate with respect to the contact which is, or is not, to be allowed between the child and any named person.
>
> [*s. 44(6) (a)*]

Directions can also be sought (and challenged) *after* the EPO has been made.

Not only must the authority, in the absence of directions to the contrary, allow contact with the child, but also it must, if it accommodates the child, "endeavour to promote" such contact "unless it is not reasonably practicable or consistent with his welfare" [*Sched 2, para. 15*].[4] This makes it all the more important to settle the issue when the EPO is granted. This could pose considerable problems for fieldworkers. Clearly they will not want to risk an adult absconding with the child (for example, from a hospital ward) or injuring him or her on a visit, but it may be difficult to make a convincing case to a magistrate that their fears justify refusal of, or strict control over, contacts. As an alternative the authority (which acquires parental responsibility on the making of the EPO) could seek a Specific Issue Order or a Prohibited Steps Order (see p. 26–7), but this will involve significant legal input. The fear that difficulties might arise over parental contact, necessitating time-consuming court appearances, may discourage fieldworkers from seeking EPOs. One way around this problem, at least in urgent cases, may be for the authority to ask the police to take the child into "police protection" (see p. 93). In such a case, contact with the child need take place (if at all) only to the extent that the relevant police officer considers that it is both reasonable and in the child's interests [*s. 46(10)*]. But a child cannot remain in police protection for longer than seventy-two hours and, if forcible entry is required, it will be necessary to apply for an EPO in any case (see p. 93). These difficulties could make the alternative of seeking a Child Assessment Order (see p. 90) more attractive to fieldworkers.

Duration of EPOs and application for their discharge

Section 45(1) has adopted the Working Party's recommendation that EPOs should last no longer than eight days. (If the eighth day is a Sunday or holiday, the order will expire at noon on the next day.) The period can be extended by seven days (this can be done only once) if the magistrate

> has reasonable cause to believe that the child concerned is likely to suffer significant harm if the order is not extended.
>
> [*s. 45(5)*].

No appeal can be brought against the making of, or refusal to make, an EPO, or any directions made in an order. However, once a child has been held under an EPO for seventy-two hours, the child, the parents, anyone with "parental responsibility" for the child or anyone with whom he or she was living immediately before the order was made may apply to a court for it to be discharged [*s. 45(8) & (9)*]. But they cannot do this if they were given notice of the hearing at which the EPO was made and attended it. Nor can they appeal against an extension of the order. Nevertheless, local authorities must be prepared for many challenges being made after the seventy-two hour period expires. It will become very important for social services departments to call in the local authority legal department as a matter of routine immediately an EPO is obtained. The lawyers will need to assemble the evidence and documentation in readiness for any challenge to the order. The inadequacy of the legal advice and representation available to social services departments played a significant part in both the events in Cleveland and in the death of Jasmine Beckford. Child care law is now too complex to rely on the amateur interpretations and advocacy of even experienced court officers in social services departments.

Where sexual abuse is suspected, it is advisable to move from an EPO to an Interim Care Order (see p. 95) as soon as possible. This is because the process of investigation is unusually difficult in such cases. The parents are likely to find the allegations particularly difficult to cope with, and investigation may involve specialist interdisciplinary teamwork. Very careful consideration needs to be given to whether or not it is in the child's interests to be removed from home during this process. An Interim Care Order is more flexible than an EPO which is designed to deal with the protection of a child in immediate danger.

Who may apply for EPOs and procedural requirements?

Although *anyone* may apply for an EPO, this will, in practice, normally be done by a social worker acting on behalf of a local authority social services department. If someone else does it (for example, an employee of the NSPCC), the social services department must be informed. Applications are likely to become more formal. The extent of the change will become clear only when new Rules of Court made under *section 52* of the 1989 Act are published. Although the rules of evidence will not apply [*s. 45(7)*], it is expected that the applicant will be required to give evidence on oath and support it by a written statement, either submitted at the time of the application or within twelve hours afterwards. The magistrate (who may hear the application anywhere) will have to record in writing his or her reasons for making or refusing the order. These will be supplied to the parents (and the child, where this is possible). The magistrate has a duty to appoint a guardian ad litem for the child "unless satisfied that it is not necessary to do so in order to safeguard his interests", and the magistrate may appoint a solicitor to represent the child [s. 41(6)(g)]. Since an EPO is intended to be only an emergency measure for a limited period, these appointments should not routinely be necessary. They are likely to complicate relations between parents and local authorities and, if frequently made, would place great strain on the supply of guardians who, it seems, could achieve little before the EPO lapsed. Of course, if there is a question of long-term measures affecting the child and the family, care proceedings are likely to follow and a guardian and solicitor will properly be required (see pp. 115–17).

It is unfortunate that the controversy aroused by the use of Place of Safety Orders in the exceptional circumstances of the Cleveland case may have led to an unnecessary degree of legal formality being introduced into an emergency procedure, to the possible detriment of the safety of children.

Child Assessment Orders

Apart from any directions which might be part of an EPO, social workers have no power to require parents to produce a child for medical examination simply because they feel uneasy about her or his condition. It was in order to strengthen the hand of fieldworkers that it was proposed that the Child Assessment Order (CAO) should be created. After considerable uncertainty as to their necessity, or even desirability, these provisions were introduced at a late stage in the Parliamentary progress of the Bill on the instigation of the Association of Directors of Social Services and the NSPCC.

The court (probably a single magistrate) may make a CAO if satisfied that (1) the applicant has reasonable cause to suspect that the child is suffering, or is likely to suffer, significant harm; (2) an assessment of the child's "health or development, or of the way in which he has been treated" is necessary to establish if the suspicions are well founded and (3) it is unlikely such an assessment can be satisfactorily made without a CAO [s. 43(1)]. Only a local authority or an authorized person (the NSPCC) may apply for a CAO.

Unlike an EPO, a CAO can be made even if there are no reasonable grounds for believing that the child is likely to suffer significant harm *if not moved or kept from his or her home environment*. But since there must be reason to believe that the child is suffering, or is likely to suffer significant harm, the distinction is a fine one. Probably it lies in the immediacy of the threat. If the danger to the child is seen as real, but at some distance, a CAO may be more appropriate.

Although the successful applicant for a CAO does not acquire parental responsibility, as happens under an EPO, the consequences of the two orders can be very similar. "Any person who is in a position to produce the child" falls under a duty to "produce him to such person as may be named" in a CAO and to comply with such directions relating to the assessment of the child as the court thinks fit to specify in the order [*s. 43(6)*]. These could include requiring adults to participate in the assessment and keeping the child away from home if necessary for the assessment. If this is done, the order "shall contain such directions as the court thinks fit with regard to the contact that he must be allowed to have with other persons while away from home" [*s. 46(10)*]. As in the case of an EPO, a child of sufficient understanding may refuse to submit to any examination.

A CAO can last for no longer than seven days. This is a severe limitation upon its likely effectiveness in allowing assessment of certain conditions, particularly where psychiatric assessment is required or where it is unclear whether a failure to thrive is due to human or natural causes. The order cannot be extended and a second application cannot be made before six months from the expiry of the order without first obtaining leave of the court [*s. 91(15)(e)*]. If the evidence establishes that further orders are necessary to allow the assessment to be completed, we see no reason why the court should not grant permission, but these requirements could be time-consuming and obstructive. The better course would be to apply for an Interim Care Order. It is unfortunate that this time limitation on CAOs could impel the authorities unnecessarily towards more elaborate measures.

EPOs and CAOs compared

Clearly an EPO is the appropriate order if a child is in obvious immediate danger. But most cases are not so clear-cut. The initial interventive stage will probably serve two purposes. One may be to discover more about the child's condition; the other may be to induce appropriate parental conduct. Either may be achieved by negotiation without revealing (or deciding) which coercive measure might be used should voluntary co-operation fail. It is expected that attempts at a voluntary solution will be made. In case of failure, the EPO can probably be obtained more quickly than a CAO because it can be granted simply on application of the fieldworker, whereas in the case of the CAO, notice of the application must be served on various people, such as the child's parents, anyone with whom the child is living, the child him- or herself, and even someone in whose favour a Contact Order is in force. Considerable time might pass while these people are notified and obtain legal representation. A guardian ad litem may be appointed. Furthermore, if a CAO is granted, there is a risk that it may be appealed to the High Court (this cannot be done for an EPO). There is a certain absurdity in having such an elaborate procedure for an order that cannot last for more than seven days. But an EPO, too, will carefully have to be prepared, especially if medical examination is sought and if it is considered that contact between parents and the child should be restricted, otherwise it may face challenge after seventy-two hours. The strangeness of the greater procedural formality surrounding the CAO is accentuated when it is remembered that its effects will usually be less drastic than an EPO's. Nevertheless, it is hard to see that fieldworkers should not acquire the result they wish, if their evidence supports it, by using a CAO instead of an EPO. There is the added advantage that the order can be granted without needing to show that the child's safety demands immediate removal from home. Against this must be set the short time-span of the CAO. But the EPO lasts only a day longer (though this may be extended by a further seven). Despite this, the more elaborate hearing and the risk of appeal, fieldworkers may prefer the more flexible CAO to the EPO, hedged around as the latter is with technicalities, except where the child's removal is urgently necessary. They may find that the service of notice of the application on a parent by itself produces the desired result.

As a precaution, courts are empowered to make an EPO even if the application is for a CAO. It is difficult, however, to envisage on what basis a court could make such a substitution unless new evidence available after the application for a CAO has caused the applicant to decide that an EPO is preferable.

Police protection

As an alternative to an EPO, the police will continue to have power to remove children into a suitable place or prevent their removal from a hospital or other place if there is reasonable cause to believe that the children will suffer significant harm if this is not done [*s. 46(1)*]. They must inform the local authority and take such steps as are reasonable to inform the child's parents, everyone with parental responsibility for the child and anyone with whom the child had been living. The police do not acquire parental responsibility over the child, but they must do "what is reasonable in all the circumstances of the case for the purpose of safeguarding or promoting the child's welfare (having regard in particular to the length of the period during which the child will be so protected)" [*s. 46(9)*]. No child can be kept in this way for more than seventy-two hours, but the police can then apply for an EPO without necessarily informing the local authority [*s. 46(7) & (8)*]. Parents, people with "parental responsibility", those with whom the child had been living, anyone with a right of "contact" with the child (or anyone acting on behalf of these) should be allowed to visit the child, but only if the police (or local authority, if the child is accommodated by it) think this is "both reasonable and in the child's best interests" [*s. 46(10)*].

Although authorities will be reluctant to turn to this procedure because the introduction of the police (for example, to prevent parents' removing a child from a hospital ward) may aggravate an already difficult situation, the new formalities surrounding EPOs may make this route more attractive in emergencies than it was in the past. But these powers do not entitle the police to enter premises without a warrant (see p. 95) except under their general powers to prevent breaches of the peace and serious crime.

No power to remove adults

Although attempts were made to introduce a power for the forcible removal of adults from premises, fieldworkers do not have such power and there is no machinery for them to acquire it. A spouse or cohabitee can, however, bring proceedings in either the county court or the magistrates' courts asking for the exclusion of his or her partner if this is demanded by the child's interests. This is a matter for that individual and will require specialist legal advice. But fieldworkers should know that if they think that an adult is ill-treating (or is likely to ill-treat) a child and that adult is *willing* to leave the home, the authority may assist that person to obtain alternative accommodation and make cash payments towards this [*Sched 2, Pt. 1, para. 5*].

No powers of forcible entry

These emergency powers have one very important limitation. Although the report of the Kimberley Carlile inquiry recommended that social workers should have the power to enter and inspect premises, this has not been accepted.[5] If it had been, the result would be a substantial shift in the present balance between personal freedom and state supervision. Although the use of such a power might save some children from harm, its existence might seriously threaten the voluntary relationship between social workers and their clients which allows them to work together in the interests of many more children.

An EPO on its own does not allow anyone, even the police, to enter premises against the wishes of the occupier. But, if requested, a magistrate can specifically authorize the applicant to enter named premises and search for the child covered by the EPO, or another child who may be in danger on the premises [*s. 48(3) & (4)*]. Anyone intentionally obstructing someone who has been authorized to do so from entering and searching commits an offence [*s. 48(7)*]. But it will not come naturally to most social workers to flaunt these powers in the face of a hostile or reluctant householder, and in such a case they will probably ask for help from the police. The presence of a police officer telling an obstructive person that they may be prosecuted if they refuse entry will probably be enough to gain admission, but if the householder continues to refuse entry, the social worker will have to go back to court for a warrant which will authorize the police to assist by enforcing the entry and search using reasonable force if necessary, and may direct (if the police officer chooses) that he or she be accompanied by a doctor, nurse or health visitor [*s. 48(9), (10) & (11)*].

Under the previous law, a police officer could not enter premises without a warrant even to take a child into "police protection". The 1989 Act contains no provision for police warrants and the old provision giving magistrates the power to grant a warrant to a police officer forcibly to enter premises to search for and remove a child has been repealed. If, therefore, the police are refused entry to a house, or part of it, and believe that a neglected child is inside, they will have to apply for an EPO with a warrant to enter.

There are special provisions penalizing the improper removal of children who are under an EPO or in police protection, and for their recovery [*sections 49 and 50*]. Fieldworkers should obtain legal advice in such circumstances.

Interim Care Orders

Quite frequently neither the local authority nor a child's parents will be in a position to present their full case to the court after the short time in which the child can be held on an EPO. But the child can continue to be held only by order of a court. If a local authority wants to continue to hold a child, *or if it wishes to continue a process of investigation which does not necessarily involve keeping the child away from home, but where parental co-operation cannot be assured*, it will have to apply for an Interim Care Order. By this stage the legal process is becoming fairly advanced, and we shall explain the place of interim proceedings in Chapter 8 when we consider the steps taken in preparation for the presentation of a case before the court. Nevertheless, it must be stressed that a full Care Order need not be the inevitable outcome of interim proceedings. *Protecting Children: A Guide for Social Workers undertaking a Comprehensive Assessment*, published by the Department of Health, advises fieldworkers about the factors they should consider in an investigation, including the desirability or otherwise of removing the child from home during this time.[6]

Notes

1. *Cleveland Report*, paras. 16.12–13.
2. See *House of Commons, Standing Committee B*, 23 May 1989, col. 221 (Mr Mellor).
3. See the discussion in *House of Commons, Standing Committee B*, 13 June 1989, col. 574 *et seq.*
4. The duty to "promote" contact applies only if the authority is "looking after" the child [*Sched 2, para. 15*], which includes children "provided with accommodation by the authority in the exercise of any functions (in particular those under this Act) which stand referred to their social services committee under the Local Authority Social Services Act 1970" [*s.22 (1) (b)*]. This includes children held on an EPO in local authority

accommodation, but not those retained elsewhere, e.g. in a hospital, under an EPO. But in either case contact must be allowed if sought (subject to direction to the contrary).

5. *A Child in Mind: Report of the Commission of Inquiry into the Circumstances Surrounding the Death of Kimberley Carlile*, London Borough of Greenwich, 1987.

6. *Protecting Children: A Guide for Social Workers Undertaking a Comprehensive Assessment*, London: HMSO, 1988.

Chapter seven

Grounds for bringing care or supervision proceedings

Under the old law the grounds upon which a local authority could pass a resolution assuming parental rights and a court could make a Care or Supervision Order were quite different. It is not necessary to examine these differences in detail, but, in general, the grounds for a *resolution* tended to refer to *deficiencies in the parents* (or their death or absence), whereas the grounds for an *order* referred to the *state of the child*. The new law was intended to combine these provisions. This task was made easier by the fact that *in practice* care proceedings tended to be less concerned with the state of a child (which was often undisputed) than with the reason why he or she came to be in that state. In effect, the dispute was often about whether the parents were responsible for the child's condition and, if they were, whether this was due to such inadequacy or recalcitrance on their part that the state ought to intervene.

The primary grounds

The grounds for court intervention were redrafted to reflect this reality. They now run as follows:

(a)   that the child concerned is suffering or is likely to suffer significant harm, and

(b)   that the harm, or likelihood of harm is attributable to

(i)   the care given to the child, or likely to be given to him if the order were not made, not being what it would be reasonable to expect a parent to give to him; or

(ii)   the child's being beyond parental control.

[*s. 31(2)*]

These conditions require elaboration. The following points are of particular importance.

The child must be under seventeen (or sixteen, if married) [s. 31(3)]

Conditions (a) and (b) are cumulative: both must be proved in a particular case before the order is made

The harm must be "significant"

The legislation offers some guidance as to how "significance" might be assessed:

> Where the question of whether harm suffered by a child is significant turns on the child's health or development, his health or development shall be compared with that which could *reasonably be expected of a similar child.* (Emphasis added.)
> [*s. 31(10)*]

What this means is that, particularly when courts assess the effects of neglect, the child's development will be charted in accordance with standard developmental criteria, such as those prepared for the DHSS by Mary Sheridan.[1] These usually categorize children by age, but the statutory test requires courts to take into account factors specific to the child, such as physical or mental handicap.

The relevance of past and anticipated future harms

The original version of the Bill, following the old law, would have permitted the authority to prove that the child "has suffered" significant harm. This was later dropped in favour of the expression "is suffering" because it was felt that this might allow intervention simply because the child had suffered harm in the past which was unlikely to be repeated.[2] The point is weak, because proof of the ground does not of itself permit the making of the order (see p. 105). Furthermore, a child is unlikely to be actually suffering the harm complained of when the court hears the application. It will therefore be necessary for the courts to adopt the common-sense interpretation employed with respect to the expression "his proper development is being avoidably prevented" under the previous law. It was held that that expression referred to the point of time immediately before the process of protecting the child concerned is first put in motion.[3] Furthermore, when looking at that point of time, the court could *also* look to the events of the past and, in a hypothetical way, to the future, because a child's development was a continuing process. In the same way, we suggest that under the 1989 Act the court is concerned to construct a picture which will show whether, at the point of time immediately before the first intervention to protect him (whether by application for an EPO, CAO, Care Order or Supervision Order) the child was *in an environment* in which he or she was then suffering significant harm. This would allow evidence of past harms as well as the child's present condition and the prognosis for the future.

In practice, the fact that the 1989 Act expressly allows evidence of anticipated harm will mitigate most problems of interpretation. It is bound to be part of the authority's case that the child is at risk of future harm, and no doubt evidence of past harm can be used to support this claim. Where the 1989 Act departs significantly from the previous law is that it *also* allows a case to be brought on the basis of anticipated harms *alone*. This innovation had been the subject of considerable debate. Some people felt that it was unsafe to give magistrates such far-reaching powers. If intervention on such a speculative basis were to be permitted at all, they thought that this should only be sanctioned by judges in wardship proceedings. But a comparable power had been available since 1968 in Scotland under the administration of Children's Panels which had fewer procedural safeguards than magistrates' courts (*Social Work (Scotland) Act 1968 s. 32(2)*). Even the previous English law allowed the juvenile court to intervene in some cases of anticipated harms, such as when harm had already been caused to another child in the same household, or where a resolution had been passed on the ground of parental unfitness. It is the merger of care proceedings and the procedure for assuming parental rights by resolution which has made this change inevitable. A local authority can no longer prevent a parent reclaiming a child it is looking after under a voluntary arrangement by passing a resolution assuming parental rights. But the authority may believe that it would be unsafe to return the child into the environment offered by the parent, even though the child has not actually suffered harm in the past. The authority can now argue that there is a likelihood of significant harm occurring as a result of an anticipated failure of parental care.

It remains to be seen how courts will react to applications brought in these circumstances. Under the earlier law the court had to decide whether the parent was of such "habits and mode of life" as to be unfit to care for the child. It is possible that a parent might have fitted this description even though he or she would not have been likely to cause the child significant harm (an example might be a religious recluse).[4] Under the new law the authority will need to specify the kind of harm which it anticipates that the child is likely to suffer as a result of the parent's character or lifestyle. Only experience and judicial interpretation will establish *how* likely the harm must be. The courts will probably say that the harm must be "more likely to happen than not", but this could be unduly restrictive. The degree of risk to be accepted should, surely, also reflect the severity of the harm which might be caused.

Nevertheless, a local authority would, for example, be able to make a case for refusing to return a child to a parent whose mental condition represented a potential threat, whatever that parent's actual experience of caring might be. The most difficult decisions are likely to arise where an authority is asked to return a child who has not actually been ill-treated. The authority has to balance its overriding duty to protect the interests of children against the general social expectation that parents should normally bring up their own children. In coming to a decision, the authority should keep in mind the more flexible range of orders, incorporating different degrees of supervisory power, which can now be made if the need for intervention is proven (see p. 134).

There has been some speculation as to whether intervention should be allowed on the birth of a child on the sole basis that the mother had failed to observe recommended antenatal care. Under the previous law, the House of Lords decided that intervention was permissible in a case where the mother had abused drugs during her pregnancy.[5] In that case both parents had continued to be addicted to drugs after the birth. Although decided under statutory words that have been repealed by the 1989 Act, it is probable that a similar conclusion could be reached under the new provisions. However, the express reference in the new Act to the *likelihood* of the child's suffering significant harm will allow the court to concentrate more directly on what will be the central practical matter: will the child be at risk if he or she is allowed to be brought up by these parents?

Lack of reasonable parental care

It is not enough simply to show that a child is suffering significant harm, or is likely to do so. There may be many causes for this, from disease to congenital handicap or social and environmental factors, such as under-nourishment due to poverty or disability due to atmospheric pollution. Child protection law is not designed to solve these problems. Its purpose is to monitor the manner in which people with "parental responsibility" for the child exercise that responsibility. Parents can work only within the environment in which they find themselves. There are many things which they cannot reasonably be expected to change and which should be tackled by other social programmes rather than by interfering in the parent–child relationship.[6]

This explains the new requirement introduced by the 1989 Act that the harms to the child must be attributable to the care given (or likely to be given if the order were not made) "not being what it would be reasonable to expect" a parent to provide for any child in a particular context. (As an alternative, it could be shown that the child is beyond parental control: see p. 104.) In deciding what care it would be reasonable to expect a parent to give, the court has to focus on the circumstances in which the care-givers (they need not be the natural parents) in the actual case find themselves and ask: what would a reasonable parent have done? The circumstances must include the whole environment as well as the attributes of the child. In the original draft of the Bill, the reference point was to be what it would be reasonable to expect the parent of a "similar child" to give him or her. This was changed in Committee to "such a child" and, at Report stage, simply to "the child" in question. But, as there was no discussion of any of these amendments, it is unclear whether they were considered substantial or merely technical.[7] If they were intended to modify the implication that the parent's conduct should be seen in the light of behaviour common to parents of children in the same social or ethnic group, they should have been fully debated. In any case, we think that deciding what it would be reasonable to expect of a parent of the child in question necessarily requires taking into account the parent's social and cultural milieu.

Some people may object to such relativistic evaluations. It is true that if everyone in the street neglects, or assaults, their children, that is no reason not to take action against some of them. But care proceedings are not an instrument of social change. They cannot remove poverty or alter deep-seated cultural practices (even assuming they should be altered). They represent *one particular form* of state intervention in family life: the forcible acquisition of responsibility for a child by the state because the standard of care being offered falls substantially short of what his or her parents should be offering. There are harms which will always justify intervention. Reasonable parents cannot be impervious to the values of the wider community in which they and their children live but, in principle, it is right that family failure, and the extent to which the harm it causes justifies compulsory intervention, should be assessed against the background of the environment in which it occurs. It must be left to the good sense of the courts to draw the line. If it is thought to be too difficult, as in controversies over corporal punishment or ritual mutilation, it may be for Parliament to provide guidance. Otherwise, to put the matter briefly and brutally, there would be little to stop the forcible removal of children from the homes of the destitute on the grounds of poverty alone.

What happens where a child suffers because a parent is of very low intelligence, or is psychologically disturbed? The question for the court is whether the standard of care being given, or likely to be given, is below that which it would be reasonable to expect *a parent* (of such a child) to give; not whether it would be reasonable to expect it of *this* parent. At first sight, this might seem hard on parents. A parent's failure to give adequate care may be due to some accident of fate – a mental illness, mental handicap or severe physical disability – rather than wilful neglect. It is difficult to *blame* a parent in such circumstances. But if that parent fails to make locally acceptable alternative arrangements for the care of the child, or refuses voluntary help from health or social services, and the child suffers significant harm, or is likely to do so, intervention would be permissible. The child's basic right to a certain standard of care overrides whatever excuses or justifications that might be offered by or on behalf of a parent.

Emotional development and delinquency

Some people have argued that assessments of emotional and psychological development are so subjective that compulsory intervention should be restricted exclusively to cases of proven physical harm. The Working Party rejected this view. "By 'development' we mean not only his physical progress but also his intellectual, emotional and social or behavioural development, so that it is clear that a child who is failing to learn to control his anti-social behaviour as others do is included" [*Review Report*, para. 15.14]. The 1989 Act reflects this approach:

"harm" means ill-treatment or the impairment of health or development;

"development" means physical, intellectual, emotional, social or behavioural development;

"health" means physical or mental health; and

"ill-treatment" includes sexual abuse and forms of ill-treatment which are not physical.

[*s. 31(9)*]

These definitions raise a number of questions. We can foresee two distinct types of case arising under the heading of emotional or behavioural harm. In the first, the effect of parental conduct towards the child (perhaps sexual abuse, or acute indifference, the so-called "Cinderella syndrome") may cause emotional harm to the child, shown by withdrawal, failure to socialize or other behavioural symptoms. In these circumstances, the case for intervention is as straightforward as in relation to physical damage. But an impairment of social or behavioural development might also be displayed through delinquent or anti-social behaviour by the child. Will this be grounds for bringing care proceedings? The Working Party thought that it might [*Review Report*, para. 15.27].

The effect of taking this view is to retain the approach which inspired the Children and Young Persons Act 1969 and its attempt to decriminalize juvenile delinquency. Criminal behaviour was seen as merely a symptom of some developmental injury. This approach was abandoned by the incoming Conservative Government in 1971 but left a legacy in the form of the old statutory procedures, which had been designed to deal with child delinquents and were in practice used almost entirely for children who needed protection against others. The 1989 Act generally attempts to redesign the system to fit child protection or child care goals and sharpen the contrast with legal and institutional responses to delinquency. The persistence of the 1969 approach seems inconsistent with this.

There might be fewer problems about including delinquents within the new provisions if it were also always necessary to show that their misbehaviour was due to inadequate parental care (although it would be extremely hard to show a positive connection between the deviance and the parental failure). This situation would at least share a common element with the usual child protection cases, namely, a lack of proper parenting. But the new grounds may also be satisfied even if there were no inadequacy in the parents if it is proved that the child is "beyond parental control". Even the best of parents might lose "control" over a child.

Our point is not that such forms of misbehaviour should not be subjected to some kind of control. But we would be concerned if "developmental harm" were interpreted as including behaviour where the child's misdeeds *towards others* activated intervention motivated by their protection, rather than focusing on the actions of others *towards the child* and his or her protection. Where misbehaviour takes the form of provable offences, it should be dealt with in a manner appropriate to the offence. The child's general social background should be relevant only in deciding the appropriate penalty. *Section 90* goes some way towards this by removing the power of courts to make Care Orders when children have been found guilty of criminal offences. But if the child's behaviour falls short of the criminal, unless there is clear evidence of both parental unfitness and developmental harm *apart from the fact of that behaviour*, it seems inappropriate to use child protection law to control that conduct.

Alternatively, that the harm, or risk of harm, is attributable to the child's being beyond parental control

Under the previous law, care proceedings could be brought simply on the ground that a child was "beyond the control" of a parent. This is no longer possible. However, if the requisite degree of harm to the child can be shown, or shown to be likely, compulsory powers can still be obtained even if the harm is not due to a failure of reasonable parental care but because the child is beyond parental control. We have already criticized above the possible use of these provisions in relation to delinquent children. However, they may properly justify intervention if the child was at risk, for example, as a result of drug abuse.

The court is not bound to make an order

We observed earlier (p. 83) that, even if an authority believes that a child might be suffering (or about to suffer) significant harm, it is not *bound* to take specific action, and we expressed our reservations about this apparent dilution in the authorities' duties. Once an authority does launch care proceedings, the reformers wished to cling to every chance that compulsory intervention might be avoided, and set up a final hurdle to be crossed before a Care or Supervision Order could be made. The court cannot make an order "unless it considers that doing so would be better for the child than making no order at all" [s. 1(5)].

This provision is very similar to the "care or control" test under the earlier law, whereby a court had first to consider whether the child was in need of care or control which he would not receive if the order were not made. It had little effect in practice because courts seemed to assume that where a child had been proved to have suffered harm, the child would not receive the care he or she needed without an order. But the new provision is likely to have more impact because it is anticipated that the new procedural rules for care proceedings will require the authority to reveal to the court its plans for the child once the order is made. The court will then need to evaluate these proposals and decide whether (1) they *need* an order to be implemented and (2) they will improve the child's situation in any case.

The court must remember the "check-list"

It will be recalled that *section 1(3)* sets out a "check-list" of factors to be taken into account whenever a court makes certain orders (see pp. 31–2). *This also applies to orders made in care proceedings* (and, indeed, to their discharge) [s. 1(4) (b)]. In practice, the factors in the list will inevitably be covered in the local authority's case, but perhaps it is worth emphasizing that "the ascertainable wishes and feelings of the child concerned (considered in the light of his or her age and understanding)" appears first on the list.

What has happened to the other grounds for intervening under the 1969 Act?

The circumstances under which care proceedings could be brought under the old law also included the child's being exposed to "moral danger" and of being of compulsory school age and not receiving proper education (the truancy ground). These provisions no longer appear in the new law. How are such situations now to be dealt with?

Moral danger

The origins of this provision lay in Victorian legislation which attempted to prevent juveniles from acquiring delinquent values by associating with known criminals or other persons of ill-repute. In modern times it has been almost exclusively concerned with attempts to prevent the sexual exploitation of girls. It is a crime for a man to have sexual intercourse with a girl under sixteen, but where the man is himself very young or the girl's behaviour is more generally disturbed, it may not be appropriate to deal with the offence by means of a prosecution. The Working Party did not specifically discuss this type of case, but its view seems to have been that unless harm was caused or was likely, legal intervention, at least regarding the child, was not justified. It seems doubtful whether sexual promiscuity by a child can be considered *in itself* to cause, or to be likely to cause, "significant harm", unless the authority was willing to attempt an assessment of the risk of the child's contracting AIDS or other venereal infections. The evidence in such a case would probably have to turn on an assessment of the impact on the child's emotional development or mental health rather than simply the fact of sexual precocity. There might be some difficulty in proving parental failure or lack of control where parents are aware of a voluntary sexual relationship involving teenagers and condone it, although it should still be possible to cover those cases where parents are forcing daughters into prostitution. In general, the same arguments would apply to boys engaged in sexual activity, although the law has rarely been used to protect them except where the relations are homosexual.

Truancy

The Working Party realized that a child might be failing to attend school as required under the Education Act 1944, and yet not satisfy the "harm" test of the new legislation. For this reason, local education authorities have been given the power to bring a new and distinct type of proceedings for a Education Supervision Order. The authority need show only that the child "is of compulsory school age and is not being properly educated" [*s. 36(3)*].

If it is felt that the child is, or is likely to be, suffering such harm that care proceedings would be more appropriate, this can be done only by the authority's social services department, to whom the education authority should refer the case. The case will now turn around a review of the child's intellectual development rather than the mere fact of school non-attendance.

Notes

1. Mary D. Sheridan, *The Developmental Progress of Infants and Young Children*, DHSS, Reports on Public Health and Medical Subjects No. 102, London: HMSO, 1960.
2. See *House of Commons*, Standing Committee B, 23 May 1989, col. 221 (Mr Mellor).
3. *D. v. Berkshire County Council* [1987] 1 All ER 20 at 33 (Lord Brandon).
4. *Lothian Regional Council v. T.*, [1984] SLT 74 (Sheriff Court, Scotland, interpreting the identical Scottish provision).
5. *D. v. Berkshire County Council* [1987] 1 All ER 20.
6. In a case reported from Greater Manchester in November 1987, three babies previously born to a particular couple had all died within their first year of life. No medical cause could be found for their deaths. When the mother again became pregnant, the social services committee decided that the new baby should be removed at birth (unfortunately, however, the mother subsequently suffered a miscarriage). Given the medical history, there was probably a "likelihood" of significant harm occurring to the newborn child if it returned home and that it might have been in the child's interests to have remained under hospital supervision during its first year. But, at least in the absence of further evidence than that revealed in the newspaper reports, it did not appear that the parents failed to provide a proper standard of care. If this was so, compulsory intervention would not be possible under the new law.
7. See *House of Commons, Standing Committee B*, 23 May 1989, cols. 220–30 and *House of Commons Debates*, 27 October 1989, vol. 158, col. 1323. The lack of discussion could indicate that the amendments were thought to be merely technical.

Chapter eight

Preparing a case

This book is intended to explain new legislation rather than to discuss administrative arrangements. However, the new framework will have implications for the pattern of relationships which has developed since the early 1970s to co-ordinate the efforts of the various public and private agencies involved in child care. Although local authority social services have been given the leading role in this area, many children's problems will first be identified by other agencies. Any legal proceedings by social services will normally follow discussions between people from the various services involved with a family. The local authority will depend heavily on evidence provided, and probably presented, by staff from other agencies.

Case conferences

Nature and purpose

The most important forum for the discussion of a case and the best way to deal with it is likely to be the case conference. There may be preliminary meetings between representatives of various agencies, if, for example, an immediate decision has to be made about the discharge of a child from a hospital ward or to seek an Emergency Protection Order. In a serious case, however, the stage will be reached when a formal conference concerning the child will need to be convened. This will normally be the responsibility of the social services department, although some authorities have delegated the role to the NSPCC. (Where this has happened, authorities ought to review the arrangements in the light of the new Act's stress on the primary role of social services departments to ensure that their statutory responsibilities can be met.)

The central functions of a case conference are to bring together information, to evaluate it, to advise social services about its implications and to obtain a commitment to their decision from the other agencies concerned. It is essential to remember that any decision for or against legal proceedings is the sole responsibility of the social services department and that the role of other participants is advisory. This is why we believe that conferences should be chaired by a social work manager of sufficient seniority to make decisions on behalf of the department and to carry authority in reminding other participants of the proper extent of their contributions.

The *Cleveland Report* recommended[1] that parents should be invited to attend case conferences unless the Chairman thought this would make it difficult to give proper consideration to the child's interests. We think this reflects a common misunderstanding of the role of case conferences. They are not pre-trial reviews of the case where an adversarial testing of the evidence might be appropriate. A better analogy might be with the "conference" between ordinary parties in civil litigation and their legal advisers, where the strength of a case and the available evidence are reviewed and a decision taken about how best to proceed – by seeking further information, by negotiation or by pressing the matter to trial. No one would dream of suggesting that plaintiffs should have the right to sit in on defendants' conferences or vice versa.[2]

There is a similar misunderstanding in *Working Together* (para. 5.45), where the DHSS gives special attention to the importance of involving parents in decision-making, citing recent opinions from the European Court of Human Rights that failure to provide for this might be in breach of the European Convention on Human Rights and Fundamental Freedoms. But those cases were concerned with decisions being made *after* children had come into care (see p. 142) and have no bearing on the preparation of applications which will go to a court hearing where parents will have a full opportunity to challenge them as the Convention requires.

If parents want to state their views to the case conference, there is no reason why they should be denied the opportunity to do so. What is important is that the conference treats this as part of the evidence on which it will reach its decision, rather than having parents remain to participate in the discussion of others' evidence and turning itself into a kind of alternative court. *Working Together* (para. 5.46) also points out that it is important, where practicable, that the case conference should be aware of the views of the child or children concerned. Depending on the circumstances of the case, this might be achieved either by having the child attend in a manner similar to that of the parents or by having a social worker or some other person speak on the child's behalf.

The importance of legal advice

The analogy with a client's conference with their lawyer underlines the significance of adequate professional legal advice at case conferences. Indeed, its absence was one of the gravest shortcomings of the procedures reviewed by the Cleveland inquiry, although the panel itself failed to recognize the omission.[3] If it is felt that compulsory measures may be necessary, case conference members must have a realistic appraisal of their legal position. Otherwise they may decide to go forward and fail, with the risk that parents will then cease to co-operate with the child care services on a voluntary basis and the child will lose such protection or support as this makes possible. Conversely, case conference participants may fail to realize the strength of their own case and falsely conclude that it is too weak to present to a court, despite their concern. Even if the evidence really is weak, a legal adviser may be able to suggest ways of strengthening the case or propose alternative legal means of achieving the desired objectives.

The appropriate source of advice is the legal department of the local authority. In some areas, child care cases are done at arm's length by the legal department, leaving the preparatory work to a courts section in the social services department. This section may acquire considerable *ad hoc* expertise, but this is not comparable to the wider knowledge of law, procedure and the skills of advocacy that a lawyer can usually contribute. The complexity of the new legislation will underline the gulf between the practical knowledge of courts section staff and the professional training of a solicitor. Many authorities have already expanded and reorganized their legal services so that a lawyer is available to attend every case conference and to supervise the preparation of a case, if the social services department decides to proceed to court. This seems much more desirable from all points of view – children, parents, staff and courts – as a way of ensuring that cases have a proper legal basis and are presented in a professional manner.

The main problem has been the rather high turnover of young and inexperienced solicitors in local government legal departments. Child care work has been seen as having relatively low status and little relation to advancement for local government solicitors. However, those departments which have created social services support sections and offered some opportunities for career progression and creative litigation do not seem to have had such severe staffing problems. Those authorities which have not previously adopted this method of working should take the opportunity of the new legislation to review their current practice and to consider whether it is adequate to meet the new circumstances. They may need to be encouraged in this by central government if the 1989 Act is to realize its objectives.

As employees of the local authority, the lawyers may feel obliged to pursue a case which they believe to have little chance of success, if they are so instructed by social services. But social workers should also appreciate that lawyers will be concerned not only about their professional reputation but also about the authority's longer-term relationship with its local courts if they are asked to bring proceedings with poor evidence or inadequate preparation. There may be a few circumstances when concern is so substantial that a case should be brought even if the direct evidence is thin, but these have to be the exception rather than the rule. On these occasions, of course, the court may be more disposed to respond to the concern, if it is accustomed to hearing well-organized and cogently documented presentations.

Outcome of case conferences

If the conference decides that further action is necessary on the case, it must consider at least the following issues: (1) that a key worker for the case has been properly identified; (2) whether the child's name should be placed on the Child Protection Register; (3) whether (further) legal proceedings should be brought; (4) whether, in a case of suspected sexual abuse, a Specialist Assessment Team, as recommended in the *Cleveland Report*, should be involved (if it has not already been); (5) a plan of future action for the case and (6) informing the parents (and, where appropriate, the child) of what is proposed.

In what follows we assume that a decision has been taken, on proper legal advice, to seek a Care or Supervision Order as the appropriate intervention mechanism. The use of other legal procedures, such as wardship or Section 8 Orders (see Chapter 2) involves more complex legal expertise and should be used only where sound legal reasons indicate that care proceedings would be inappropriate.

Choice of court

Under the previous law, applications for a Care or Supervision Order could only be made to a magistrates' court. As we have explained (pp. 37–8), under the 1989 Act the Lord Chancellor, may, by Rules of Court, permit such applications to be made also in the High Court or in a County Court, although both he and the Solicitor-General have said that care proceedings will be initiated in magistrates' ("Family Proceedings") courts, with unusual cases being transferred to a different level of court. There are no compelling reasons for routinely using other courts. The central issues to be decided in these cases normally concern assessments of the level of child care acceptable to the community and of the aptitude of the parents as caregivers. We do not believe that the professional judges of the High Court and County Courts are necessarily better able to make such evaluations than the lay members of a magistrates' court. Indeed, magistrates may well be in closer touch with community values on these matters than judges.

Apart from such considerations, local authorities are likely to favour magistrates' courts because legal costs would be lower. Nevertheless, cases of unusual complexity might be better dealt with at a higher level. It is a matter on which the legal department will need to make the necessary judgment.

Interim Orders

In many cases, the child might already have been made subject to an EPO or CAO. As we have seen (pp. 85–92), these are of limited duration. Care proceedings do not necessarily have to follow the obtaining of an EPO. Other forms of intervention might suffice; indeed, the mere fact that the order has been used might have been sufficient to "bring the parents to their senses". Nevertheless, it is clear that the making of such an order will require some rapid decision-making by the authority for, unless an Interim Care Order can be obtained within eight days from the issue of the EPO (unless in exceptional cases a seven-day extension is acquired), the child must be returned (see p. 88).

An Interim Care Order is, as its name suggests, a temporary, or holding, measure. To obtain it, the applicant must present evidence that there are reasonable grounds for believing that the conditions for making a Care or Supervision Order (discussed in Chapter 7) exist [s. 38(2)]. The advantage in having an Interim Care Order is that it has the effect, while it is in force, of conferring on the local authority full parental responsibility for the child. This will allow the authority to conduct a full diagnostic assessment of the child, although the court making the order will have power to make specific directions about this, including a direction *prohibiting* such assessment, and a child who is old enough to do so may refuse to consent to such assessment [s. 38(6) & (7)]. The court also has power to make an Interim Supervision Order. This does not confer parental responsibility on the applicant (which will usually mean that the child cannot be moved) but may contain directions regarding medical or psychiatric examination of the child (see p. 135).

Of necessity, the evidence produced at this stage, both for the authority and for other participants, may often be scanty. Even if a guardian ad litem for the child has been appointed (see p. 116), it is very unlikely that the report will be available. Other forms of written evidence may not yet have been prepared for, as we shall see, the production of such evidence has been made subject to special rules, which will extend the time for its preparation (see p. 118). Nevertheless, the authority must be prepared to produce some evidence of the "harms" or "likely harms" and of the responsibility of the parents for these. If the application is contested, the court will have to evaluate the strength of the concerns about the child, but must remember that the applicant's case need not be fully established at this stage so it should avoid a prolonged argument.[4]

An Interim Care or Supervision Order can last for anything up to eight weeks. This period may well be necessary in order to allow all participants to prepare their case, and the guardian ad litem to investigate the matter. The authority can apply for a further Interim Order or Orders, but these cannot delay the final hearing for more than four weeks beyond the original eight weeks [s. 38(4) & (5)]. Under the previous scheme it sometimes happened that witnesses

113

came to court, expecting a full hearing, only to be turned away because a further Interim Order had been agreed. This was very frustrating. The new legislation attempts to avoid this by allowing the initial Interim Order to run for a longer period than previously, although the effect of this is somewhat weakened by the fact that (at least if it follows an EPO) the order must have been made more swiftly in the first place. One of the prices to be paid by allowing more people to participate in care proceedings is that they may take longer to prepare. If it is likely that a further Interim Order will be made, lawyers and fieldworkers should alert their clients and witnesses to this and so prevent unnecessary annoyance.

One reason for possible delay should be mentioned. Sometimes authorities (and other participants) are reluctant to go ahead if criminal proceedings are pending against the parents. It is thought that they may infringe the parents' "right of silence" respecting the prosecution. But the outcome of the care proceedings is strictly irrelevant to the criminal case. There may be a slight risk that the parents' answers in the care proceedings will become known to the police and indicate how they might respond at the criminal trial, but the child's interests in rapid conclusion of the care proceedings outweigh this.[5] The 1989 Act expressly provides that no one can escape answering questions in case proceedings simply because the answers might incriminate them or their spouse. But it also prevents such answers being used against the person making them in later criminal proceedings (except for perjury) [*s. 98*].

Participants

Parties

As they were originally constituted, the only parties to care proceedings were the local authority and the child, although parents were given limited rights to participate in the hearing. The reason for this strange arrangement was that the structure of the hearing was built on the assumption that most cases would involve children who had engaged (or were alleged to have engaged) in delinquent activity. It then made sense to see the children as being "brought before the court" by the authority, given a chance to explain their behaviour and then, if the court thought it appropriate, be committed to local authority care. However, it became more common for the procedure to be used in child abuse and neglect cases than for delinquency cases, and there of course the child is in a very different position. Attempts to modify the procedure to bring it better into line with the realities of these types of case led to great complexity, and the Children and Young Persons Act 1986 for the first time made parents "parties" to the case. The reformed law now rationalizes the situation.

As we have seen (p. 44), it will usually be the local authority which initiates the proceedings. *Section 93* leaves the definition of parties to the Rules of Court which will be published later. But the Government has stated that the child, the parents and anyone whose legal position could be affected by the proceedings will be entitled to party status (*White Paper*, para. 55). So it is likely that the Rules will entitle anyone who has or is seeking legal responsibility for the child, such as step-parents, grandparents, or the father of an illegitimate child, to party status; of course, if they are *not* seeking responsibility for the child, but would simply like to express a view, they may still do this, but will not acquire party status.

A person with "party" status in legal proceedings has certain advantages. The most obvious is that he or she may be legally represented at the hearing. As far as the parents are concerned, one important result is that they will be entitled to apply for legal aid. This will be granted on the basis of their means and an assessment of the strength of their case. It would be most unusual for legal aid not to be granted in care proceedings if the parents satisfied the financial tests. The parents' lawyer will of course represent them throughout the hearing, but will also have an important part to play in the pre-hearing procedures, which we shall explain later (pp. 117–18). Finally, the fact of being a party brings with it the right to challenge the decision by appeal (see p. 149).

Guardians ad litem and solicitors

Although, as we have observed, the child is a party to a hearing, certain special considerations apply. If the child is too young to instruct a solicitor, how is legal representation to be obtained? The solution that has been found is to route this through the "guardian ad litem". Guardians ad litem are normally social workers or probation officers whose names appear on a panel administered by local authorities. They may be retired or working part-time, but may also be in employment, often with a local authority, sometimes with a voluntary agency. However, the person appointed must not be connected with the local authority which is taking part in the proceedings. They are expected to bring their own independent judgement to the case. The 1989 Act creates the basis for a framework for administration of guardian panels by regulations to be made by the Secretary of State [*s. 41(7)*].

Section 41(1) requires the court (in magistrates' courts, this in effect means the court clerk) to appoint a guardian ad litem for the child in applications for Care or Supervision Orders

> unless satisfied that it is not necessary to do so in order to safeguard his interests.

In the past it has been shown that there were very wide variations between regions in the readiness of courts to appoint guardians ad litem.[6] This may partly be due to their limited availability. But the clerk has a very wide discretion. On one occasion the parents complained to the High Court that the clerk had failed to appoint a guardian in a case where the child had been admitted to hospital, undernourished and neglected, and with multiple bruising and bite marks. The judge decided that, although there was "quite a substantial argument" for appointing a guardian in this case, he could not say that the clerk had acted "unreasonably" (and therefore unlawfully) in failing to make the appointment.[7] Nevertheless, the Government has indicated its expectation that under the 1989 Act guardians will be appointed in about 90 per cent of cases.[8] As we have seen, the 1989 Act contains similar provisions for the appointment of guardians on application for EPOs and CAOs. Since these will be short-term measures, we are doubtful of the value, or efficacy, of appointing guardians routinely in these situations.

The guardian is not supposed to act as an *advocate* for the child in court, but rather to investigate the case by speaking to the relevant social workers, reading the social services' file on the case, interviewing the parents and, where possible, ascertaining the child's views. To assist guardians in these duties, they have been given the right to "examine and take copies of" local authority records which are relevant to the case [*s. 42(1)*].

Under the previous system, the guardian was required to instruct a solicitor to appear *for the child* in court and there is no reason to believe that this will be changed. (The parents may instruct their own solicitor.) The child's solicitor should be drawn from the local "child care panel" of lawyers set up by the Law Society. The major duty of the guardian is to present a report of his or her investigations to the court. Guardians will, however, work closely with the child's solicitor and provide him or her with any necessary information and may give evidence in the witness box. But their reports are submitted to the court, and copies must be sent as rapidly as possible to all the parties to the case.[9] Rules of Court to be made under the 1989 Act will be able to specify further ways in which guardians can be required to assist the courts. (See also *s. 41(9)*.)

If, however, the child is old enough to instruct a solicitor, he or she has the right to do so, and in that case the child's right to appoint and instruct the solicitor overrides the right of the guardian, although of course the guardian can still submit a report and appear as a witness. Whether a child is old enough for this purpose might have to be decided by the clerk or magistrate at the pre-hearing. If no guardian is appointed, the court may appoint a solicitor to represent the child if it thinks this would be in the child's best interests and the child is able and willing to give instructions [*s. 41(3) & (4)*]. Since a very young child will not be able to instruct a solicitor, this means that such a child will go unrepresented unless a guardian is appointed. Since it can rarely be in a child's interests (no matter how young) that it is not represented at all in proceedings to which it is a party, the implication seems to be that a guardian should be appointed in all cases unless the child is old enough to be able to instruct a lawyer personally.

The preliminary hearing

Some changes introduced in the new legislation have meant that care proceedings have become more complicated than they used to be. This has led to the introduction of a new stage in the procedure, called the *preliminary hearing*, which will usually have to take place at some time between the making of an Interim Order and the full hearing. Some juvenile courts had already introduced such a procedure in order to try to reduce delays.

One of the purposes of the preliminary hearing will be to fix a timetable for the course of the proceedings, such as the dates for the full hearing. It will be important for everyone concerned to be there to ensure that appropriate dates are chosen.[10] But the preliminary hearing will also provide the opportunity to resolve problems that may have arisen in the preparation of the case.

When making the application, or shortly thereafter, the local authority will need to inform the parents of the grounds for its application and give a brief statement of the facts on which it intends to rely. It will also have to provide copies of the statements made to them by witnesses on whom it intends to rely. This may all take a little while to prepare. The new rules are also likely to require the authority to indicate the nature of the order it is seeking and, in general terms, what it plans to do with the child. Having received this information, the parents (or their lawyer) and the guardian ad litem (if appointed) or the child's lawyer will assess what to do. They may wish to acquire more information. Previously the magistrates' court had no power to compel the authority to provide any. It is intended that the new procedures will give the guardian ad litem special privileges in this regard. The persons opposing the application (usually, the parents) will also be required to give their reasons for opposing it (*White Paper*, para. 57).

Clearly any of these issues may be contentious, and one function of the preliminary hearing is to allow the court (in the person of the clerk or a single magistrate) the opportunity to settle any dispute that may have arisen over these preliminary matters. Rules of Court will be made dealing with the procedures to be followed at preliminary hearings [*s. 93(2)(e)*].

We shall discuss questions of evidence later (pp. 122–8), but we should notice that the preliminary hearing procedure will have an important part to play in the way evidence may be assembled for the hearing.

Notes

1. *Cleveland Report*, p. 246.
2. In *R. v. Harrow London Borough Council, ex parte D.* [1989] 2 FLR 51, a High Court judge held that an authority had not acted unfairly in refusing to invite a mother to a case conference which resulted in the children's being placed on the At-Risk Register.
3. *Cleveland Report*, paras 10.30, 10.31. See also J. Rea Price "The Cleveland Report – A Social Services' Perspective", (1988) 1 *Child Law*: 4–5.
4. *R. v. Birmingham City Juvenile Court, ex parte Birmingham City Council* [1988] 1 All ER 683.
5. See *R. v. Inner London Juvenile Court, ex parte G.* [1988] 2 FLR 58; *R. v.*

Exeter Juvenile Court, ex parte H. (1988) 18 *Family Law* 334.

6. *R. v. Plymouth Juvenile Court, ex parte F. and F.* [1987] FLR 169.
7. See the *Plymouth* case, note 6 above.
8. *House of Commons, Standing Committee B*, 23 May 1989, col. 255 (Mr Mellor).
9. *R. v. Epsom Juvenile Court, ex parte G.* [1988] 1 All ER 329.
10. See Ian Young, "Care Proceedings: Pre-hearing Reviews", (1989) 19 *Family Law* 366.

Chapter nine

Presenting a case

This chapter will outline the present approach of juvenile courts to questions of evidence in care proceedings. The 1989 Act gives the Lord Chancellor power to make regulations governing the way care proceedings will be conducted under the new system and these may alter the way evidence is used in them. Nevertheless, it is likely that some control over legally admissible evidence will be retained, and it will be helpful to fieldworkers if we consider some of the problems of translating professional judgements into legally admissible evidence which have been faced under the old system and how these may be dealt with under the new one. It should be stressed that what follows applies essentially to proceedings for Care or Supervision Orders (including Interim Orders) and CAOs. Different considerations apply to hearings for EPOs (see p. 89).

Witnesses

Anybody who works in the field of health and social welfare may find themselves in court as a witness. This involvement will usually follow from their statements at a case conference or to members of the social services department who are working up a case to go to the local authority's lawyers. If called upon to do so, local authority employees must give evidence as part of their conditions of employment. The same compulsion does not apply to former employees or contractors, like foster-parents, or to employees or contractors of other agencies, most particularly the health services. If somebody refuses to become a witness, however, the court does have the power to issue a witness summons at the request of a party to the proceedings requiring them to give evidence. The request will be made at the preliminary hearing (see pp. 117–18).

Most doctors are prepared to volunteer evidence but health visitors, on the advice of their union, prefer to be served with a witness summons. This allows them to emphasize to families their independence from the local authority and the fact that their evidence is being given under the court's compulsion. General practitioners could also find this to be a helpful procedure, although we would express some scepticism about whether many families really understand the difference. Failure to respond to a summons is contempt of court and a grave matter. Anybody committing such an offence can expect a substantial fine, and the court even has power to order their imprisonment.

The power to apply for a witness summons is not, of course, confined to the local authority. It may be used by the child's representative and the parents. This can occasionally be a source of some embarrassment for agency staff who find themselves summonsed to appear, in effect, against their service's case. People like fosterparents, in particular, may find their position rather awkward, since local authorities are often reluctant to jeopardize their goodwill by asking them to appear, and they may find the first indication of their involvement when a summons drops through the letterbox. This is very often not something they have bargained for as an outcome of a desire to offer some voluntary service to the community in fostering. What is important to remember is that this is a *court* order. The justices are responding to information given to them about someone who is believed to have evidence which will help them determine the case but who will not come forth voluntarily. The order directs the witness to attend and give evidence *to* the court rather than *for* a party.

It should be remembered that relevant information acquired in the course of the doctor–patient relationship does not have any special legal protection. Doctors may sometimes seek to evade the apparent conflict between their commitment to medical confidentiality and their duty to the court by saying that the child, not the parent, is their patient, and that the information was acquired in the course of their treatment of the child. While this will often be true, it may not always be the case. For example, a psychiatrist may have information about the parent's mental state acquired while treating the parent which is relevant to the child's home situation. This should nevertheless be made available to the court.[1] Furthermore, in November

1987, the Standards Committee of the General Medical Council expressed the view that if a doctor believed that a child was being physically or sexually abused, not only was it permissible for the doctor to disclose that information, but also the doctor was under a duty to do so.

Although the doctor–patient relationship is not protected in law, protection is given to the local authority and the NSPCC in so far as this is necessary to allow them to shield the identities of their informants.[2] It would not, therefore, be possible to require the local authority (or an officer of the NSPCC), either before the hearing or by questioning during the hearing, to reveal the names of any person who may have reported the case to them.

What are rules of evidence?

It has been said that the rules of evidence are no more than common sense written carefully. Nevertheless, many people, especially social workers, express great concern about the way their evidence is treated. They often feel that the issues they are dealing with are too vague to satisfy the strictness of legal tests. There is some truth in this at the level of attitudes: lawyers do sometimes give social workers an impression of being dissatisfied with evidence that seems to be based too much on feelings and intuitions and too little on facts. Certainly, lawyers are also inclined to discount social work evidence in favour of medical evidence, especially, but not exclusively, in cases of abuse or neglect. Doctors are considered to make much more impressive witnesses.

There are good reasons for this. Medicine and law have a long-established relationship with fairly well-developed conventions and ground rules. Social work is a much more recently created occupation whose tasks and approaches are poorly understood. At the crudest, few lawyers will ever be social work clients while most will be doctors' patients. Moreover, medicine and law have certain conceptual similarities in that they both tend to adopt a rather positivist view of the world. Both are inclined to act as if truth were simply a matter of grasping the right set of external facts. Social work has been much more influenced by relativist philosophical currents which tend to see both "truth" and "facts" as rather problematic, not to be seized once and for all as a basis for dogmatic statements.

Social work and legal judgments, then, are rather different. Fieldworkers build up their picture of a family from a variety of sources. This picture is continually subject to revision and re-assessment. The credibility of the basic data can be tested against the worker's personal experience of the family, its kin and its neighbourhood. If necessary, the data can be systematically checked. A court of law cannot do this: reality is assessed at one time for all, like a snapshot. It thus becomes of utmost importance to develop rules, built up over years of experience, which guide courts as to exactly how much credibility should be given to evidence coming from different sources. The court does not have the fieldworker's advantage of instinctive feeling for differentiating the value of various sources. It must act solely on what is said before it in the courtroom. In that context, some forms of evidence will inevitably be considered better than others. The law of evidence is primarily concerned with apportioning the weight which is to be given to each item.

Facts, hearsay and opinions

Ideally, decisions in court should be made on the basis of factual evidence given by witnesses from their own observation or participation in the events under review. In the nature of things, this is not always possible. The law, then, has to deal with other categories of evidence, of which the two most important in care proceedings are hearsay and opinion. Hearsay is where a witness relates what someone else said about X as evidence of the truth of X: for example, where a social worker recounts a neighbour's telling her that he had seen a child being hit as evidence that the child had been hit. Opinion is where witnesses draw their own conclusions from facts about which evidence may or may not be directly given: for example, where a health visitor infers from fluctuations on a child's weight chart that a child is being underfed while at home. Courts are cautious about hearsay evidence because the person whose statements are related cannot be cross-examined on them. They are also wary of statements of opinion, partly because the facts upon which the opinion is based may be equally as shielded from questioning as hearsay evidence and partly because it can be said to be the role of the court, rather than of witnesses, to draw conclusions from facts.

But, while experience has taught the law to be cautious about those categories of evidence, they are not totally excluded. Over the years, a set of rules has been developed which specify the conditions under which such evidence may be admitted and the precautions which must be taken in its use. These rules were substantially liberalized by the Civil Evidence Acts 1968 and 1972, but these Acts do not apply in the juvenile court. Under the 1989 Act, regulations may be made abrogating or modifying the hearsay rule in care proceedings [*s. 96(3)*]. If the models of the previous Acts are followed, we might expect an approach like the following to be adopted.

Case records

The "hearsay rule" applies to what is written as much as to what is said, so a document recording certain facts should not be admitted as evidence of those facts unless the person who wrote it can be questioned about it in court. But a strict application of this rule would fly against common sense. Why should we not accept the written record of a casualty department concerning the medical condition of a patient, even if the officer who compiled it has now disappeared? Similarly, the high turnover of social work staff would make social work records vulnerable if the original compiler had to be called in every case they were needed as evidence. It is likely that such written evidence will now be admissible if its author was under a duty to keep the records and acted on information supplied by someone with personal knowledge of the facts alleged. This does not of course mean that their content has to be believed; simply that it forms part of the evidence.

Statements

Under the previous law, a witness was allowed to report a statement made by a parent, or other person who had had "charge" of the child, if what was said indicated something about the person who made the statement.[3] So a social worker, or even a neighbour, could stand in the witness box and say: "She told me she had struck the child". If the court believes this, it can be treated as evidence that she had, indeed, struck the child. Of course the mother will be there to deny it, if she wishes. But it is important to remember that the same rule does not apply if the parent (or person in similar position) had been heard to say: "His father beats him". The words must refer to the person saying them, not someone else. Also, statements of third parties could always be admitted if their relevance was not to prove the truth of what they asserted, but the mere fact that they were made. For example, it would be proper to report that someone said: "I am Napoleon", not as evidence that he was, but because it says something about his state of mind at the time. Similarly, a fieldworker could report that, for example, a wife complained of her husband's conduct, not as proof of the truth of those allegations, but as evidence of the state of the marital relationship.

These rules have some merit, but, even if they are retained, the new regulations are likely to make them even more flexible. Sometimes reports of what someone may have said on an earlier occasion could be important, such as a nurse's remarks about the condition of a child which she made on examining it, or what a neighbour said about the behaviour of a parent. These would strictly be excluded as hearsay. But, provided that the nurse or the neighbour is called as a witness, and this is notified to the other parties to the case, there is no reason why such evidence should not be used. The party calling the witness would "put it to the witness" that they had made the reported statement, which they could then affirm or deny.

The hearsay rule has caused particular difficulty with regard to statements by children. If a witness says that a child has complained that he or she has been sexually abused, the child's statement is hearsay and cannot be used as evidence that the child had made the statements.[4] The extension of the Civil Evidence Act 1968 to care proceedings in juvenile courts would not change the position much because that allows the evidence to be admitted only if the person who made it can be called to give evidence on oath.[5] A child cannot do this unless he or she understands the nature of the oath. It is likely that the power to alter the hearsay rule in care proceedings will be exercised to allow the court to take notice of such reports, at least when supported by unsworn evidence given by the child or by other forms of direct evidence. *Section 96(2)* of the 1989 Act allows a court to hear a child's unsworn evidence if the child understands he or she must tell the truth and has sufficient understanding to justify the court hearing it.

Agreed evidence

The parties may agree evidence, which may then be submitted in writing to the court. The most obvious example of this is medical evidence. A medical report may not be in dispute, yet strictly it should not be admitted unless the doctor who made it is in court to answer questions about it. One reason for this is that medical reports often contain matters of opinion, and the person whose opinion is given should be available for cross-examination (see p. 123). However, often all the parties agree to accept the medical diagnosis, and, if they do, the new regulations will confirm current practice that this can be submitted in writing. However, it is important to ensure that when such an agreement is made, which will be at the preliminary hearing, the court takes care that a party who is not represented appreciates what he or she is agreeing to permit.

Opinions and experts

As with hearsay, the law does not seek to exclude opinion but simply to ensure that it is carefully appraised. It is recognized that the dividing line between questions of "fact" and of "opinion" is not always easy to draw. The statement "The car was being driven fast" is partly a statement of fact but also partly an inference from those facts as to their cause and their normality. Similarly, statements like "The child showed signs of disturbance" or "The child looked under-nourished" combine both factual observation and evaluative comment. So long as there is an underlying basis of fact for such observations, no court will take objection if anyone were to make such statements, although the witness can be expected to specify in more detail, if asked, the factual basis for the observation.

There is, however, a degree beyond which such evaluations pass from what one may call "common-sense" interpretations to rely upon a more global assessment by the witness. For example, general statements like "The child is in need of psychiatric help" or "This parent's behaviour is likely to cause lasting physical or emotional damage to the child" draw heavily upon the witness's theories about child development and predictions about future behaviour. In principle, such statements should be allowed only if made by people considered competent to make them, so-called "expert witnesses". There is a good deal of misapprehension among fieldworkers, and some lawyers, about what the legal position in relation to experts really is. It seems, for example, to be thought sometimes that there are precise rules designating which categories of professional person are or are not to be considered "experts". This is not so. In principle, a court can decide on a witness's expertise in each individual instance. In doing this it will make a pragmatic assessment of his or her qualifications and experience. Sometimes a court will be more impressed by a lay person with many years' practical experience working with children than by a newly qualified fieldworker. Whether one agrees with this or not, what should be appreciated is that there is no mystique in the rules about experts: the courts, especially the juvenile courts, respond to witnesses in much the same way as any lay person would.

What is probably more important, even, than the attitude of the court is that of the lawyers, especially those of the local authority. The lawyer is essentially operating on the same lay, common-sense basis as the magistrates, and the lawyer's primary concern will be to try to present to them the most convincing case he or she can. Most lawyers familiar with child care cases will be prepared to present a fieldworker as an "expert" if they think that he or she will impress the court. Not unnaturally they will tend to have more confidence in the more senior workers, and one cannot rule out the relevance of appearance and demeanour. But, given satisfaction on these matters, many lawyers will be prepared to ask fieldworkers questions of general opinion, prefacing the question with a statement such as "What in your professional opinion would be ...?" or "As an experienced and expert worker in the area of child care, what would be ...?" But fieldworkers should always be prepared to back up any opinions they give with factual evidence as far as they can. Any expert is open to questioning in this way. Nothing creates a worse impression on a court than an "expert" who has been exposed in cross-examination as having based his or her opinion on insufficient examination of the facts of the case.

The necessity of being able to support opinion with fact is particularly important for fieldworkers in the social services departments. By their very nature, their judgements are peculiarly liable to attack under cross-examination by an opposing solicitor or barrister. There is inevitably a greater degree of uncertainty about such social assessments than there is about more obviously scientific matters. Whether a parent's child care practices are of an unacceptable standard or whether a parent's behaviour in relation to the child is likely to improve are less easy to prove than the state of the child's body. Moreover, the facts of the child's physical condition will rarely be in dispute. For these reasons, the evidence of medical witnesses has caused many fewer problems in care proceedings. Lawyers readily admit that they like detailed medical evidence, not only of the more obvious kind where a child is physically injured, but also such as is provided by weight charts and developmental tests. In fact, some of this evidence is less obviously "scientific" than it looks, as it makes certain assumptions about the normality of child development which may not be appropriate to this particular case. Hence the desirability of obtaining information about the child in different settings in order to give a comparative dimension to any evaluation of his or her progress in the home environment.

Presenting evidence

The preceding sections have described the principles which help to determine what evidence the courts will and will not accept. Before concluding, however, we should like to note some points which can help to maximize the impact of the evidence as it is presented.

When witnesses arrive at the court building, they will be asked to wait outside the courtroom where the case is being held. It is not usual for witnesses and parties to have separate waiting areas, and this can occasionally be a source of embarrassment. If possible, witnesses should avoid any discussion of the case with other parties or their solicitors. Once the hearing begins, witnesses will be asked to come in one at a time by the usher, who is usually recognizable by a black academic-type gown. The usher takes the witness to the witness box, which in a modern court is generally more like a lectern, and administers the oath. If the witness wants to make an affirmation or take a non-Christian oath, it is as well to speak to the usher before the hearing.

Courtrooms vary a great deal in age and layout, especially when juvenile courts are sitting and there is some attempt to make them more informal. Typically, the three magistrates will sit at one end of the room, possibly on a slightly raised dais. In juvenile cases, at least one magistrate will always be a woman. The court clerk sits in front of the magistrates. The witness stand is usually to the left, as one faces the magistrates, and the dock to the right. In care proceedings, this should be empty, since they are not of a criminal nature. The lawyers may sit either side facing the magistrates. There will probably be press seats behind the witness stand, although these are likely to be empty, since reporting on juvenile cases is restricted. Finally, across the court and facing the magistrates are seats for the public.

The general public are not admitted to juvenile proceedings. Only people with a legitimate interest – other staff from the agencies involved, students and researchers – are allowed to attend, by permission of the court. Occasionally, uniformed police officers may be present on routine court duties. If they are not actually involved in the case and there is no serious prospect of disorder the court may reasonably be asked to request them to leave.

After being sworn, the witnesses will be taken through their evidence by the lawyer who has asked for them to attend. (We shall assume for the moment that this is the authority's solicitor.) Evidence has to be given by means of question and answer. If there are questions a witness particularly wants to be asked, the lawyer should be briefed beforehand. The main point to remember is that an experienced witness tries to give as full an answer as possible during the examination-in-chief. This is the occasion to make the case, and short or monosyllabic answers are useless. Magistrates often find visual aids helpful. Photographs, diagrams, weight charts and the like can all summarize technical points and save time on detailed description. When answering questions, remember that it is the magistrates who are the audience. The solicitor is eliciting a story for their benefit. This means that it is important to speak clearly and slowly enough for them to take notes, somewhere between dictation speed and conversation.

Wherever possible, a witness should try to give direct evidence. This may cover such matters as the behaviour of a child, the state of the home, the conduct of parents towards each other or whatever. It is not good enough to speak in generalities. For instance, if asked about a parent's demeanour in an office interview about financial assistance, a social worker might say: "Mr Brown was aggressive." From the court's point of view, this is opinion, although it may well be sufficient as a practical basis for casework. If, however, the social worker were to say: "Mr Brown knocked my telephone on to the floor, called me a tight-fisted bastard and threatened to punch me in the face if I showed up at his house again. From this, I concluded that he was in an aggressive mood," the court is presented with facts and an inference, which the justices can check for themselves. To give another example, a health visitor might say: "Johnny Brown was being inappropriately fed." It would carry much more force if she were to say: "I made a point of calling at lunchtime on five occasions in that six-week period. On one occasion, I saw this eight-month-old baby sharing a packet of chips with his sister. Once I saw him with a bottle of milky tea. I did not see him fed on the other occasions and could see no baby food anywhere in the kitchen. I thought this was inappropriate for a child of his age." In both of these examples, the evidence already exists in the workers' observations and reasoned inferences, both of which should, as a matter of good practice, have been fully recorded. What has to be done is to show the court that reasoning, giving both the facts and the conclusions. The court can test the inferences and decide whether the conclusion is more likely than not to be correct.

This direct evidence is much more satisfactory than relying on the hearsay reports of neighbours or relatives. In fieldwork, of course, these may well be rather important, especially as the fieldworker can check the informants' credibility in a variety of ways. If the case looks like coming to court, though, the fieldworker should always try to verify the reports by direct observation. If these reports are crucial to the case, they should be passed to the authority's lawyer with a view to calling their originator as a witness. In making a decision on this, the solicitor will want to know what sort of impression the person is likely to make in the witness box. Will the witness prove reliable under cross-examination? Is the witness vulnerable to accusations of malice, dishonesty, or even inadequate parenting of his or her own children? Any of these could damage the weight of their evidence and have a bad effect on the authority's case.

One of the features by which magistrates assess people is their general demeanour. They recognize, of course, that many witnesses are nervous, but it helps greatly to try to sound confident in what one is saying. It is no good expecting the magistrates to believe evidence if the witness sounds unsure or hesitant. On the topic of demeanour, it is also worth making some effort which shows an acknowledgement of the formal nature of the occasion. Casual dress is likely to be taken as indicating a lack of seriousness and to detract from the status of the witness as someone worth listening to.

After the examination-in-chief comes the cross-examination. This is the point at which the other lawyers (for the child, the guardian ad litem or the parents) have a chance to test the strength of the evidence. There are a number of techniques, but probably the most common are direct questions, trying to elicit information which has not previously come out, or questions which, in effect, propose alternative interpretations of alleged facts. It is here that the importance of having confidence in one's evidence becomes apparent. What the lawyer is looking for are signs of uncertainty or ambivalence, and his or her questions are likely to be designed to draw these out. The lawyer may ask a question which is phrased to obtain a simple answer when the evidence is more complex. Thus, "Are you saying that these parents are fundamentally inadequate?" invites a "Yes" or "No" answer. Either may lead into difficulty; the former because the lawyer can then go on and point to positive features; the latter because it edges away from the authority's case. Another problem that is often encountered is where the cross-examination asserts that the parents are really willing to co-operate. It can be hard for a witness to reject such offers without seeming harsh and unfeeling. The key advice is to get any reservations in first. If a question can minimally be answered "Yes" or "No", the lawyer is entitled to cut in and ask the next question once the answer has been given, even if the witness tries to go on. Rather than answering "Yes, but ...", the witness should aim for "But ..., yes."

A frequent difficulty is the cross-examining lawyer's lack of familiarity with the structure of health and welfare agencies. Health service personnel, in particular, may find themselves being asked about a child's future in care. They cannot properly answer such questions, which are entirely within the discretion of social services. It is not always easy to refuse, but the best course is for the witness to explain that this is not something they can answer on and to look to the magistrates or the clerk for directions. The expected new emphasis on social services outlining their plans for the child to the court will make it even more important for other witnesses to avoid being drawn into the discussion of matters which are not their responsibility.

One thing witnesses should not be scared of is an aggressive or hectoring lawyer. Magistrates tend not to like that sort of conduct, especially when applied to inexperienced witnesses. Quiet firmness and persistence are the hallmarks of a good advocate. The same, incidentally, is true for the local authority's lawyer. Social workers, and staff from other agencies, are sometimes disappointed by the apparently low-key nature of the lawyer's cross-examination, but this often bears much greater dividends than an aggressive attack on, say, a nervous mother, which reduces her to tears and forfeits the magistrates' sympathy for the authority. Occasionally, the magistrates may themselves ask questions, as may the clerk.

After cross-examination, the authority's lawyers may re-examine to clarify any ambiguities which have emerged. This is usually very brief, and the witness can then step down. Witnesses may remain in the court for the rest of the hearing, and must certainly not leave the building without the magistrates' permission. The reason for this is that a witness may be recalled at any point, if new material arises in subsequent evidence and the court wishes to reconsider what has previously been said. In practice, this is extremely rare and the courts are reluctant to detain people unnecessarily. If a witness does not want to remain to the bitter end, it is best to mention it to the relevant lawyer, who will then request the witness's release after the examinations have been completed.

In the past fieldworkers have often felt unduly hesitant in considering the suitability of their evidence for presentation in court. They seem to think, especially in cases of emotional neglect, that the kind of evidence available to them will be inappropriate, either because it does not have a sufficiently 'scientific' character or because they will not be regarded as having the status to make 'expert' statements. No professional should be deterred from taking appropriate action for these reasons. It is certainly true that practitioners should be careful to record their observations in the manner suggested above, and be prepared to put their judgements on as substantial a basis as possible. Careful attention to detail will frequently enable this to be done. It is for the lawyer to "translate" this evidence into its legally acceptable form. If thoughtful and experienced fieldworkers are convinced of the need for court action to protect a child, then, provided that the grounds fall within the scope of the legislation, there should rarely be any strong reason why a case should not be assembled which, from a purely evidential point of view, could respectably be presented to the court.

The guardian ad litem's report

A guardian ad litem can give evidence as a witness, in which case the position is as discussed above. But the guardian's report can contain material which falls outside the rules of evidence. The 1989 Act makes it clear that a court can draw its own conclusions from the contents of the report [s. 41(11)]. At present, the guardian's report is read by the court only once it has decided whether the case has been established according to the evidence presented in the normal way. This may change under the new system if the authority's plans for the child's future will need to be unfolded to the court as part of its application for an order. The guardian's report may then be revealed at any earlier stage, enabling the court to have before it a wider sweep of material on which to make its decision. But in such circumstances, the guardian could expect to be cross-examined on the contents of the report.

Notes

1.   *Report of the Review Panel appointed by Somerset Area Review Committee to consider the case of Wayne Brewer*, Somerset Area Review Committee, 1977.
2.   *D. v. NSPCC* [1978] AC 171.
3.   *Humberside County Council v. D.P.R.* [1977] 1 WLR 1251.
4.   *Bradford City Metropolitan Council v. K. (Minors)*, *The Times,* 18 August 1989.
5.   *H. v. H. and C.* [1989] 3 All ER 740.

Chapter ten

The outcome of care proceedings

If an authority has applied for a Care or Supervision Order, the court may, of course, make one of those orders. This chapter will focus on their implications. However, it must be remembered that the reformed legislation also allows the court to make a Residence Order, a Contact Order, a Prohibited Steps Order or a Specific Issue Order in care proceedings. These orders were described in Chapter 2. The court cannot make a Residence or Contact Order in favour of a local authority [*s. 9(2)*]; so those orders can be made only in favour of a person (perhaps a relative of the child, or a foster-parent).

Supervision Orders

When a court makes a Supervision Order, its purpose is to allow a child's parents to retain that child at home in their care on condition that the way in which they carry out their responsibilities can be monitored by the social services department. Under the old law Supervision Orders were very weak. Because they had originally been designed as a response to delinquency, they were formally directed towards the child and few requirements could be imposed on parents.

The new legislation places the supervisor under a *duty*

(a) to advise, assist and befriend the supervised child;
(b) to take such steps as are reasonably necessary to give effect to the order; and,
(c) where
    (i)   the order is not wholly complied with; or
    (ii) the supervisor considers that the order may no longer be

necessary,
to consider whether or not to apply to the court for its
variation or discharge.

[*s. 35(1)*]

The Supervision Order may still impose requirements on the child, for example, to attend for medical assessment or treatment. But more importantly, it may now require the person with parental responsibility over the child, or any other person with whom the child is living, to ensure that the child complies with the supervisor's directions regarding, for example, attendance at a specified place (e.g. a play-group, or a clinic), or that they themselves accept parental training or guidance as directed by the supervisor [*Sched 3, paras 2 & 3*]. But there are still two important limitations. First, the supervisor cannot require the child or anyone else to undergo medical or psychiatric treatment. If desired, this will have to be built into the Supervision Order itself, and, if the child is of sufficient understanding, his or her consent will also be necessary [*Sched 3, paras 4(4) & 5(5)*]. Second, the order cannot impose requirements on adults without their consent [*Sched 3, para. 3*], although such consent is likely to be offered by many parents involved in care proceedings as a way of "buying off" the possibility of having the child removed under a Care Order.

While there may clearly be cases where supervision is preferable to the greater disruption of a Care Order, social workers, and indeed, courts, should be wary about being drawn into a kind of "plea bargaining" where a Supervision Order is seen as a "compromise". The local authority should have considered the possibility of supervision during the course of its preparation of the case and, if this was rejected at the time, it should resist being thrown off course by courtroom negotiations. A Care Order does not necessarily commit the authority to removing the child from home for a long period, or even at all. But it provides the authority with the strongest possible lever with which to bring pressure on parents to modify undesirable behaviour patterns or dangerous living arrangements.

Supervision Orders can be seen as only temporary measures. If improvement is not achieved relatively swiftly, a more permanent solution may be indicated. So a Supervision Order must terminate after one year, although it may be extended to a maximum of three years. Nor may requirements be imposed on the child or the parent as to exceed ninety days [*Sched 3, paras 6 & 7*].

It should be remembered that a Supervision Order in itself does not confer on the supervisor any right to enter the parents' home without their permission in order to examine the child. If the order contains a provision that the supervisor should visit the child (which would surely be routine), and the supervisor is refused admission and wishes to force an entry, he or she will need to apply for a warrant authorizing a constable to assist [*s. 102(6)*]. If the supervisor wishes to remove the child, he or she must apply for and use an EPO (see pp. 85–90). The supervisor may of course return to the court if a condition is broken. The new Act has, however, made it significantly more difficult to alter the supervisor's powers. If a Supervision Order has failed to achieve its objectives, or worries about a child persist, the old law allowed the court to replace it with a Care Order without having to establish the intervention ground again. Now, both local authorities and parents will need to go through all the costs and stress of re-hearing the original evidence. If there are reasonable doubts about the prospects of a Supervision Order being workable, fieldworkers should apply for a Care Order, even if it is administered initially as if it were supervision. A local authority cannot be made to accept a Supervision Order without its agreement [*Sched 3, para. 9*] but a refusal could have very serious implications. Such a decision should be taken only after consultation at a high level in the social services department.

Care Orders

The new legislation states that

> where a care order is made with respect to a child it shall be the duty of the local authority designated by the order to receive the child into their care and to keep him in their care while the order remains in force.

[*s. 33(1)*]

In addition, the authority acquires parental responsibility for the child except that it cannot alter the child's religion, consent to the child's adoption or appoint a guardian for the child [*s. 33(6) (a) & (b)*]. Nor may anyone cause the child to be known by a new surname, or remove him or her from the United Kingdom (except for a period of less than a month) without the consent of *everyone* who has parental responsibility or the permission of a court [*s. 33(7) & (8)*].

Do the parents retain *their* parental responsibility? Under the old law, they did not, and it was the original intention of the Government that "the effect of a care order is that parental powers and responsibilities are passed to the local authority and this will be specified in law" [*White Paper*, para. 35]. But the Act simply says that the local authority "shall have" parental responsibility for a child under a Care Order. Since a person does not lose parental responsibility "solely because some other person subsequently acquires parental responsibility for the child" [*s. 2(6)*], anyone with parental responsibility before the Care Order is made will retain it.

This is a significant change from the old law and could have serious consequences. Normally, as we explained on pp. 26–7, if someone with parental responsibility who is not looking after a child wishes to challenge a decision by the person with whom the child is living, he or she must apply for a Specific Issue or Prohibited Steps Order. But the 1989 Act forbids those orders being made against a local authority [*s. 9(1)*]. The result is to deprive a person who has parental responsibility of any machinery to exercise the responsibility. Not only that, *section 33(3) (b)* gives the authority the power to determine the extent to which the parent may meet his or her parental responsibility for the child.

The clear purpose of the Act is to displace the parent's responsibility with that of the authority. This is a perfectly proper objective, since the whole point of the intervention is that the parent has failed to exercise the responsibility reasonably. But the legislators have refused to take the logical step of enacting that a Care Order *transfers* parental responsibility from parent to local authority. For what can only be ideological reasons, they have insisted that the parent *retains* responsibility, but then go on to remove the means to exercise it.

This is a dangerous strategy. A parent might initiate wardship proceedings and, while the outcome is by no means certain, it is possible that the court would be sympathetic to putting that jurisdiction at the service of someone with parental responsibility. A parent might even take the Government to the European Court of Human Rights. Article 6 of the European Convention on Human Rights and Fundamental Freedoms states that "in the determination of his civil rights and obligations ... everyone is entitled to a fair and public hearing within a reasonable time by an independent and impartial tribunal established by law". If a parent retains parental responsibility after a Care Order is made but is denied the right to assert this before a court of law, it could be difficult to resist the argument that the new Act is in breach of the Convention.[1]

If either course of action were to succeed, local authorities could be faced with constant questioning of their decisions before the courts, to the detriment of the balance between authorities and courts discussed in Chapter 3. In explaining to parents their position after a Care Order is made, fieldworkers should stress that legal responsibility for the child effectively passes to the local authority.

While the authority has care of the child, it must

> safeguard and promote his welfare; and make such use of services available for children cared for by their own parents as appears to the authority reasonable in his case.
>
> [s. 22(3)]

This duty is modified only in so far as it may be necessary to restrict the child's liberty in the interests of protecting members of the public "from serious injury" [s. 22(6)]. This statement of the authority's duty seems to give it a very wide discretion in making plans for the child. Provided it believes a decision promotes the child's welfare, it appears to be able to take it. However, there are a number of constraints on the way this discretion can be used and on the kinds of decisions that can be reached.

Matters to be given "due consideration"

In making any decision about the child, the authority must, as far as is reasonably practicable, ascertain the wishes and feelings of the child, the parents, anyone with parental responsibility and anyone else (for example, grandparents) whose wishes and feelings the authority considers to be relevant [s. 22(4)]. They must give "due consideration" to those wishes and feelings (in the case of the child, having regard to his or her age and understanding) and must also give "due consideration" to the child's "religious persuasion, racial origin and cultural and linguistic background" [s. 22(5)].

We should emphasize that where this provision, and the others we discuss below, refers to a child's "parents", this includes an unmarried father even if he does not have "parental responsibility" for the child (see pp. 21–2). The extent to which an authority involves such a man will, in practice, inevitably depend upon the interest he shows in his child.

Where the child is to be accommodated

Authorities have a duty to accommodate and maintain children who are in their care [*s. 23(1)*]. *Section 20(2)* lists the ways in which authorities can accommodate children whom they are looking after. They include placing the child (in accordance with regulations) with "a family, a relative of his or any other suitable person" as well as in various types of residential accommodation. The authority must do its best to ensure that the accommodation is near the child's home and that siblings are not separated [*s. 23(7)*].

Allowing a child to go home "on trial"

Although *section 33(1)* places authorities under a duty "to keep the child in their care while the order remains in force", the same wording was used under the old law and it has never been seriously doubted that the common practice of allowing a child home "on trial" while remaining in care was perfectly proper. To be "received" and "kept" in care refers more to the abstract duty which the authority has towards the child. But, while home trials may be an important part of case management, they require careful assessment. Maria Colwell and Jasmine Beckford were killed after being returned home; Maria after discharge of the Care Order had been unopposed by the authority; Jasmine while still in care.

As a consequence of concerns raised by these types of event, regulations were made under the Children and Young Persons Act 1986, s. 1, which came into effect on 1 June 1989.[2] These were directed towards tightening management procedures when a child was returned home on trial. Before going ahead, the authority should seek the written views of various persons, including the district health authority; the person receiving the child (usually the parent) must enter into a written agreement with the authority which acknowledges that the child can be removed if the authority is not satisfied that the placement is furthering the child's welfare and sets out the arrangement for social worker visits. The authority is required to visit at intervals of not more than six weeks in the first year of the placement, and of not more than three months thereafter, and the person making the visit must "so far as practicable see the child alone on each visit". It is likely that regulations to be made under the 1989 Act will follow this model [*s. 23(5) & Sched 2, para. 14*].

Duty to promote contacts between the child and the family

Although unlike the previous law, the 1989 Act does not proclaim that the return of the child to the family is a preferred policy, it states expressly that whenever a child is "looked after" by a local authority, the authority

> shall, unless it is not reasonably practicable or consistent with his welfare, endeavour to promote contact between the child and

(a)   his parents;
(b)   any person who is not a parent of his but who has parental responsibility for him; and
(c)   any relative, friend or other person connected with him.

> [*Sched 2, para. 13(1)*]

This general directive applies to all children "looked after" by an authority, and therefore covers children it is accommodating under voluntary arrangements, or under an EPO as well as children in care under a Care Order [*s. 22(1)*]. But, in the case of children in care, it is reinforced by specific provisions which will be very important in practice. These are that

> where a child is in the care of a local authority, the authority shall (subject to the provisions of this section) allow the child reasonable contact with

(a)   his parents;
(b)   any guardian of his;
(c)   anyone who was his "residential guardian" before the order was made; and
(d)   anyone who had care of the child under the wardship jurisdiction before the order was made.

> [*s. 34(1)*]

This means that, unless the conditions set out later in the section are met, contact between the child and those persons must be allowed. Contact can be disallowed in the following circumstances:

1 If this has been authorized by the court when the Care Order was originally made. The court may do this even if the local authority does not ask for it. But it is very important for fieldworkers to think carefully about the question of contact *when applying for the Care Order* and the Act actually requires the court, before making a Care Order, to consider the arrangements the authority has made or is proposing to make concerning contact, and to invite the parties to the proceedings to comment on them [*s. 34(11)*]. The possibility that an unmarried father might turn up and seek contact ought also to be considered at this stage, to prevent the necessity of having to go back to the court later.

2 If not authorized in the Care Order, the authority may disallow contact for a period of no more than seven days "as a matter of urgency" if it is satisfied that this is necessary "to safeguard or promote the child's welfare". The Act does not restrict the number of occasions this can be done (though if it is done routinely it is unlikely to be considered a "matter of urgency") and regulations will be published specifying the procedure to be followed [*s. 34(8)*]. The authority may do this even if an order has been made requiring contact [*s. 34(6)*].

3 If the authority decides that parental contact has been unsuccessful and wishes to terminate that contact, preparatory, perhaps, to fostering the child with a view to adoption, it will need to return to the court for an order authorizing the termination. The child can also ask for this to happen [*s. 34(2) & (4)*].

The child's parents and the other persons with whom contact is to be allowed may apply at any time for an order to regulate their contact with the child. Any other person can also apply, but will need the court's permission in advance [*s. 34(3)*]. The child may make a similar application for contact with any person [*s. 34(2)*].

In further support of the presumption in favour of contact, the authority is under an obligation to "take such steps as are reasonably practicable" to inform the child's parents (and anyone with parental responsibility) of the child's whereabouts, unless the child is in care and the authority has reasonable grounds for thinking that doing this would prejudice the child's welfare. Those people should also notify the authority of their own addresses [*Sched 2, para. 15(2)*]. If a visit cannot be made without incurring the visitor in undue financial hardship, and the circumstances otherwise warrant it, the authority has power to pay relevant expenses [*Sched 2, para. 16*].

The *White Paper* (para. 64) commented rather disingenuously that the new provisions would "lead to some additional court work". Authorities must be prepared for a considerable increase in litigation over decisions about contact. Furthermore, proceedings of this kind will be very different from the initial care proceedings. These will have established harms to the child and the extent to which his or her caretakers are responsible for them. Litigation over "contact" may cover part of the same ground, but the emphasis will be more upon making judgements about the future, such as whether it is correct to suppose that the parent–child relationship will not work, or whether a satisfactory alternative arrangement can be found for this child: in short, what is the best way to promote the welfare of a child with respect to whom harm or likely harm has already been proved. As we suggested in Chapter 3, we are rather sceptical as to the extent to which the opinions of the courts on these matters (as distinct from the fairness of the procedures adopted or the reasonableness of the evidence on which the decision was taken) should be preferred to those of social services personnel.

Consultation with parents

In 1983 a Code of Practice governing the way local authorities made their decisions concerning access to children by their parents was laid before Parliament. One of its main features was the encouragement of consultation between parents and local authorities over decisions that are taken regarding their children. We have already mentioned the duty to inform parents of children "looked after" by the authority of the children's whereabouts. But the desirability of keeping parents informed extends to all major case management decisions. The DHSS Guidebook, *Working Together* (para. 5.45), also stressed the importance of "openness and honesty" with the parents. It is important for fieldworkers to appreciate that this is not only a question of good practice. It is a legal requirement as well. The European Court of Human Rights has said that, in order to comply with the obligation set out in Article 8 of the European Convention on Human Rights and Fundamental Freedoms, which demands respect for private and family life, it is necessary that parents should be fully involved in such decisions.[3] Although the Convention is not law in this country in the sense that it binds local authorities, it is likely to be taken into account by the courts if an authority's actions are challenged by judicial review.

We shall explain what is meant by "judicial review" later (pp. 146–7). At this point all we wish to emphasize is that social services departments are under a legal duty to inform parents about such decisions and to allow the parents to express their point of view. Inevitably, the extent of this duty is somewhat vague. Obviously the parents will not be entitled to be told about every detail of the child's life in care. Nor will an authority be expected to make extravagant efforts to contact a parent who has disappeared or has shown no interest in the child. It will be a question of behaving with sensible and reasonable regard to the parents' interests. This may, *in some cases*, extend to allowing the parents to present their point of view to a case conference or review dealing with the child, and to bring a solicitor with them. If the authority comes to a balanced and informed decision after having allowed the parents to make such representations, and if it has genuinely considered those representations, then its decision is unlikely to be liable to successful legal attack.

One difficult situation which may arise for the authority is where damaging allegations have been made against one or both of the parents of a child in its care, and the authority wishes to alter its plans for the child because of concerns raised by the allegations. It has been held in one case[4] that in such circumstances the authority should give the parent against whom the allegations have been made the chance to reply to them. But this might be very difficult. In the case in question, the allegation had been made by the wife that her husband had indulged in sexual perversion. If put to the husband, he might be expected simply to deny it. Yet failure to allow a parent to "state their case" could lead to a successful legal challenge to the decisions taken. Our suggestion is that where allegations of a serious nature are made regarding a parent, and social workers believe that these will affect their plans for the child, the matter should be referred to the local authority's legal department. The lawyers may then wish to raise the matter formally with the parent concerned, perhaps through his or her solicitor (if the parent has one). The authority could then proceed on the basis of the advice proferred to them by the legal department.

Restricting and punishing the child

We have explained that a local authority acquires parental responsibility of children committed to its care under a Care Order. How much power over the child does this actually give the social services? The obvious approach would be to imagine that the local authority was the child's parent and to act accordingly as common sense directed. But, although this might be reasonable as a basic rule of thumb, fieldworkers should be aware that the law has laid down some general principles and also some specific provisions.

In the *Gillick Case*[5] the House of Lords decided that a parent's rights to control the way a child behaved towards others had to be qualified by the child's own rights to take decisions for himself or herself (see p. 24). If the child had reached such an age as to understand the issues involved, and also had the maturity of judgement to deal with them, then the parent lost the legal right to impose a particular course of action on the child. Obviously this principle is open to very subjective interpretation. We can, however, be sure that any parent, and therefore any local authority to whom care of a child has been committed, can restrain very young children to prevent their endangering themselves. On the other hand, once a child reaches the age of, say, fourteen or fifteen, the power forcibly to restrain a child's movements, except perhaps in emergencies, has probably disappeared.

It might be asked how this affects the question of punishing the child. As stated earlier (p. 25), there is no law in this country forbidding a parent from exercising corporal punishment, though excessive use of this may be grounds for bringing care proceedings on the basis of the harms suffered. After corporal punishment became illegal in the state school system (see p. 25) the Government promised that corporal punishment would be forbidden in local authority children's homes, as it already is in residential care homes (where the children suffer a disability).[6] Nevertheless, it is inconceivable that children who have been committed to care should now be subjected to such punishment, certainly once they have reached school age and possibly even earlier. Foster-parents, however, even if engaged by the local authority, may not be under such a restriction.

Nor has a local authority unfettered power to lock up a child it is holding under a Care Order. The matter is controlled by regulations made under *section 25*. If it appears that the child has a history of absconding and is likely to abscond and that if the child absconds, he or she is likely to suffer harm; *or* that the child is likely to injure himself or other persons if not kept in secure accommodation, the child may be locked up. But the regulations will specify the periods for which this may be done and the period after which court authorization will be required. The child should be legally represented before the court, whose decision is subject to appeal.

If the child is not in care, these provisions do not override the basic right of a person who has parental responsibility to take the child out of local authority accommodation (see p. 77) [*s. 25(9)*].

Fostering

When a foster-parent cares for a child for whom the authority has parental responsibility, the authority retains its legal control over the child, which it may call back at any time. The authority remains responsible for all children whom it is looking after. If its staff are denied entry to premises where the children are living, a warrant may be issued to a constable to help them to enter the premises and see the children [*s. 102*].

But it should not be thought that foster-parents have no recourse to legal protection. If they have been looking after a child for three or more years they are entitled to apply for a Residence Order. If the child is in care, they may do so before three years if the local authority consents [*s. 10(5) (c)*]. If the child is not in care, and has not yet been with them for three years, foster-parents can seek the court's permission to apply for any Section 7 Order, even a Residence Order. If foster-parents resort to this frequently, there would be a risk that parents might be deterred from making use of the voluntary accommodation arrangements, so the 1989 Act states that, in this situation, unless they are related to the child, the foster-parents will need the consent of the authority [*s. 9(3)*].

A Residence Order will take the child out of care and transfer parental responsibility from the authority to the foster-parents [*s. 81(1)*]. They may also become fully involved in any legal proceedings for the discharge of a Care Order (see p. 115). However, foster-parents should be aware that once a Care Order is discharged and a Residence Order is made in their favour, the child's parents (who have never lost their parental responsibility: see p. 22) now have the opportunity to seek to impose their views on the upbringing of the child by applying to a court for a Specific Issue Order or a Prohibited

Steps Order. This puts foster-parents in a weaker position than if they had obtained a custodianship order under the old law, because those orders suspended the parental rights of anyone other than the custodians [*Children Act 1975, s. 44*]. The effect may be to discourage people from seeking to formalize their relationship with children fostered with them by the local authority unless this can be done by adoption.

Statutory reviews

Local authorities are obliged to carry out a review of the arrangements for all children who are being "looked after" by them, whether under a Care Order or otherwise. Under the previous law, this had to happen every six months. Unfortunately, it seems that many, if not most, local authorities found it difficult to comply with this duty. Under the new law, the frequency of reviews and the procedure to be followed will now be dealt with by regulations made under *section 26*.

Judicial review

We have several times mentioned a form of legal procedure called judicial review. This has developed only recently in child protection law, but is well established in other areas of administration. Essentially, it is a legal procedure through which any person with a sufficient interest in a particular administrative decision can challenge the decision in the High Court if he or she believes that it has been made improperly. An improper administrative decision might be one which is made as a result of personal bias or prejudice, or without having gone through proper procedures, or without giving the persons affected a chance to state their case. If the challenge is successful, the court's main remedy is to nullify the decision taken and to require the administrative authority to consider the question again, this time following the correct procedures.

Apart from bad cases of bias or personal prejudice, judicial review is mostly concerned to ensure that administrative authorities follow the correct procedures. This does not mean that the courts will insist on a slavish adherence to every last word of a procedural code. But serious departures from established procedures can be penalized. The courts have not held back simply because there have been no relevant written procedures, or if the procedures have been deficient. They have asserted that general principles of "natural justice" can apply in these situations and these principles will insist decisions should not be taken by people in circumstances where there is an apparent likelihood that they may be biased in the matter and that the people affected should (except in very unusual circumstances) know the gist of the decision that may be taken and be given a chance to put forward their views before it is made. These principles are very broad and their application in particular instances (for example, whether the person affected should be permitted to put forward his or her case through a lawyer) will depend on the circumstances. The best tactic is to use a common-sense approach. The more serious the matter for the person affected, the more care should be taken to ensure that the person has a full chance to put his or her viewpoint effectively.

Judicial review will not usually be available to challenge the *substance* of a case management decision which has complied with these requirements.[7] There is a chance that the person affected might argue that, although there were no procedural flaws, the actual decision was so unreasonable that no reasonable authority could reach it. This effectively requires a judge to decide that the decision was so perverse that the authority must have disregarded obvious and available evidence. It is very difficult to argue this successfully, at least if the social services department can show that it considered all the relevant information. It is important, then, not to exclude arbitrarily any item of evidence relevant to the decision in hand.

Complaints

The 1989 Act requires every local authority to establish a procedure for considering complaints made to them by any child they are looking after (and even those they are not looking after, but who are "in need") and by such children's parents, people with parental responsibility for them, anyone else whom the authority thinks has a sufficient interest in the child to warrant hearing what they have to say, and any local authority foster-parent. The complaints can, however, relate only to the way the authority looks after children. Issues concerning the investigation of suspected child abuse, the conduct of care proceedings and even contact between parents and children in care seem to be excluded [*s. 26(3)*].[8] Regulations will be published dealing with this new procedure [*s. 26(5)*].

How orders may be discharged

Unless the child concerned reaches eighteen, the effects of a Care Order can be removed only by another court order. Sometimes this is automatic, as where a Residence Order is made in someone's favour. But it will usually result from an application for its discharge by an authority, the child, or anyone with parental responsibility (it will be remembered that the child's parents do not lose parental authority while the child is in care: p. 137) [*s. 39(1)*]. Supervision Orders can be discharged in the same way, but these, as we have seen, have a limited life anyway.

There is no limit to the number of times a person may apply for discharge of a Care or Supervision Order (or the substitution of a Supervision Order for a Care Order), but, unless the court gives special leave, at least six months must elapse between applications [*s. 91(15)*]. In practice, if an applicant requires legal aid, he or she is unlikely to receive it if it appears that the procedure is being used in a vexatious manner.

We referred above (p. 139) to the fact that Maria Colwell had been killed after she had been returned home when her mother's application for discharge of the Care Order had not been opposed by the authority. For this reason, the *Review Report* and the *White Paper* took the view that the eventual discharge of a Care Order should not be made unless a court was satisfied that this would be in the child's best interests. This has not, in fact, been specifically spelt out in the Act, though it is clear the court has to give the child's welfare "paramount consideration", and take into account the check-list in *section 1(3)* [*s. 1(4) (b)*]. It must also appoint a guardian ad litem unless it is satisfied that it is not necessary to do so to safeguard the child's interests [*s. 41(6) (c)*]. Clearly the authority must produce some convincing reasons for believing that discharge of the order will serve the child's interests, but on the whole it is hard to believe that there will be many cases where the court will think that a guardian should be appointed. If there are any doubts, the court has the power to replace a Care Order with a Supervision Order [*s. 39(4)*]. Indeed, such an substitution would frequently be good practice when returning children home from compulsory care.

In the rather special circumstances where a child ceases being "looked after" by an authority (whether under a Care Order or otherwise) after reaching the age of sixteen, the authority falls under a duty to "advise and befriend" young people until they reach twenty-one if it thinks they need this and they have requested it [*s. 24*]. The advice and assistance (which can include cash) is designed to help these children to adjust to life out of care.

Appeals

Decisions made in the court system are subject to a system of appeals. The old system contained many anomalies, deriving from the fact that it was designed to deal with delinquency cases, not child protection. Appeal lay from the juvenile court to the Crown Court and the local authority had no right of appeal whatsover if it lost. The *Working Paper* (para. 6) expressed common sense when it proposed that appeals should go to a Family Court (not to the Crown Court) "should a decision be made to introduce one," and that all parties should have a right of appeal. As we have explained (p. 38) no decision has been taken over the introduction of "Family Courts" although it is intended that the existing system will be treated in a more coherent way. The 1989 Act takes the logical step in sending appeals over the making or rejection of orders by magistrates' courts under the Act to the High Court. The High Court is empowered to make such orders as may be necessary to give effect to its decision [*s. 94*]. No appeal may be brought against the making of an EPO.

Notes

1. See John Eekelaar, "Parental Responsibility for Children in Care" (1989) 139 *New Law Journal* 760.
2. Accommodation of Children (Charge and Control) Regulations, SI 2183 of 1988.
3. *R. v. United Kingdom*, Judgments and Decisions of the European Court of Human Rights, vol. 121 (July 1987).
4. *R. v. Bedfordshire County Council* [1987] 1 FLR 239.
5. *Gillick v. West Norfolk and Wisbech Area Health Authority* [1986] AC 112.
6. See *Childright* 46 (April 1988) 8 and *Childright* 52 (November/December 1988) 9–11.
7. *R. v. Hertfordshire County Council* [1987] FLR 239.
8. This is because the procedure covers only the discharge of the authority of its functions under "this Part" of the Act: *viz.* Part 3. Part 3 does, however, include the general duty to promote the children's welfare, acting in consultation with the parents and others [*s.22*]: see p. 79.

Index